CONTENTS

INTRODUCTION

An anti-inflammatory diet is an eating plan that aims to reduce or prevent chronic inflammation in the human body, which can cause many severe medical conditions if left untreated.

The diet focuses on fresh vegetables and fruits. Many plant-based foods around us give us antioxidants. It also focuses on nuts, lean proteins, whole grains, healthy fats, spices, and seeds. The intake of alcohol, red meats, and processed foods is discouraged. So you have to avoid them or limit their intake as much as you can.

Remember the following:

Vegetables and fruits have natural components known as phytonutrients, which can protect us against inflammation.

Foods that have a lot of saturated fats can, on the other hand, increase inflammation. Also, foods containing trans fats and highly processed foods can also be inflammatory to your body.

Healthy fats like omega-3 fatty acids and monounsaturated fats can help you stay away from chronic inflammation.

Also, make sure to achieve a good balance of carbs, protein, and fat in every meal you have. Your anti-inflammatory eating plan must also meet the requirements of your body by providing you with all the minerals, fiber, vitamins, and water you need.

Few simple lifestyle changes can give you many benefits. Change to an anti-inflammatory diet, get enough sleep, reduce stress, and exercise. You will certainly see a marked improvement.

You will see a reduced risk of diabetes, obesity, heart disease, cancer, and depression, among others.

The symptoms of inflammatory bowel syndrome, arthritis, lupus, and several autoimmune diseases will improve.

Inflammatory markers in the blood will go down.

Markers for cholesterol, triglyceride, and blood sugar will improve.

Your mood and energy levels will go up.

You must eat the right foods to beat chronic inflammation and avoid the diseases it causes. However, consuming only the right food is never going to be enough. You may have to make some lifestyle modifications as well.

Here are some recommendations:

Get Physical Exercise

An active lifestyle is a healthy lifestyle. Studies have shown that exercise can reduce inflammation. People who are into physical activities regularly show fewer inflammatory symptoms.

You should workout at least for half an hour a day, 5 days a week. That is a minimum. Better still if you do aerobic activities of moderate-intensity like playing tennis or brisk walking for an hour to 75 minutes or vigorous activities for 15 minutes in a day. Combine this with high-intensity muscle-strengthening activities like weight lifting a couple of days in a week.

Join a health club if you can. If you can't, then at least take up swimming classes or ride a bike to work. Don't use the escalator. Take the stairs instead. Every bit will help. Look for opportunities where you can sweat it out.

Get Enough Sleep

A lot happens when we sleep. The body repairs the organs, cells, tissues, and muscles. The chemicals that strengthen our immune systems circulate within the blood. Hormones are also made when we are asleep. Our bodies are fully repaired and recharged from sleep.

It is essential to get adequate sleep. It is very important to keep our minds and bodies healthy. According to The Center for Disease Control, 35% of all adults in the United States don't get the recommended 7 hours of sleep every night, which can be dangerous. Poor quality sleep or not sleeping long enough can cause many health hazards, including type-2 diabetes, weight gain, and inflammation.

So make sure to sleep for at least 7 hours a night. Go to bed at 11 PM. Switch off all electronics and make the room dark. Also wear comfortable clothing, ensuring that nothing is bothering you as you are trying to doze off.

Manage Stress

There are different types of stress – physical (injuries), mental (financial), and emotional (relationship issues, sense of isolation, social rejection). We are all stressed to some extent. However, there is always a negative impact on the body if the stress becomes overwhelming.

The body will lose its ability to respond if this stress is not relieved. You will begin to see the inflammatory symptoms and related diseases.

There are ways to manage stress efficiently like MBSR or Mindfulness-Based Stress Reduction, PMR or Progressive Muscle Relaxation techniques, and breathing exercises. You can also practice tai chi or yoga. Make it a habit of meditating for half an hour before going to bed. This will slow you down and help you relax. Take a break or go on a holiday if the stress seems too much.

Manage Your Weight

Obesity can be dangerous. It can cause diabetes, high blood pressure, osteoarthritis, breathing problems, gout, heart ailments, and even some types of cancer.

Research also suggests that obese people are more likely to have inflammation. Those who are overweight, especially in their abdominal area, are always at a higher risk. Adipocytes, also known as the fat cells in the belly, produce and secrete compounds, which are known to cause inflammation.

Your immune system is under pressure if you have an excessive number of fat cells. It sees the fat cells as a 'foreign invader' and tries to fight them off, which turns on the inflammatory response. This becomes chronic over time.

Luckily, even a 10% reduction in body weight will help you fight it off. An anti-inflammatory diet without sugar, little alcohol, and without red meat will help. Eating fewer calories and exercising will help you lose those extra pounds.

Avoid Toxic Environments and Allergens

To be honest, we cannot avoid toxins completely. But it will be very useful if you are aware of the environment you are in and avoid harmful materials as much as possible. This will help you reduce the inflammatory triggers.

Environmental toxins can cause cardiovascular diseases, diarrhea, chronic obstructive pulmonary disease, respiratory issues, and cancer, among others. Millions die around the world from toxins.

Food allergies can also be bad for health. Sadly, many people are not even aware of the different types of foods that can trigger allergies. So be careful. Try to identify the foods that are causing allergic reactions. Avoid them and you will see a difference. Similarly, try to avoid inhaling harmful toxins and chemicals.

CHAPTER 1: INFLAMMATION

1.1 What Is Inflammation?

Inflammation is a set of reactions generated by the body in response to an attack. This can be external like an injury, an infection, a trauma, or internal like those observed in autoimmune pathologies.

In normal times, the skin and mucous membranes help protect the body against external aggressions.But in the event of infection or injury (a burn, a wound, etc.), microorganisms (bacteria, fungi or viruses) can cross this protective barrier.This is where the inflammatory reaction comes in."It allows the total elimination of intruders and the complete repair of damaged tissue," explains Professor Ricci.

Suppose a person gets burned while preparing their meal.This awkward gesture will create a breach through which microorganisms, pathogenic or not, will be engulfed.Fortunately, cells in the immune system keep an eye on things.Among them, neutrophils and monocytes which circulate permanently in the blood arrive at the site of infection.They have receptors on their surface that allow them to recognize and fix unwanted elements.

Once contact is made, immune cells release chemical alert signals to the entire immune system.Then come other immune cells from the bloodstream.Once the last intruder has been destroyed, calm returns and the body works to repair the tissue.

The presence of visible inflammation indicates that an attack on the body has taken place, whether it is bacterial, traumatic or linked to another cause.It can happen that the inflammation is discovered only during the realization of a biological assessment, faced with signs of fatigue orunexplainedpain.Research of the origin of the inflammation must, therefore, take place to adapt the treatment of its cause.

What are the symptoms of inflammation?

Inflammatory reactions are triggered in order to defend the body against an attack.When they are visible, they manifest themselves classically by 4 clinical signs: redness, pain, swelling and increase in local heat.It can be a cutaneous or subcutaneous inflammation (abscess, erysipelas, shock).When the inflammation is internal, these signs exist but are not visible.Only the pain is felt, often increased in intensity during the night.

What are the signs of inflammation in the blood test?

Inflammation is biologically characterized by an increase in reactive protein C or CRP, the rate of sedimentation and the number ofwhite blood cells.This reflects the establishment of the body's fight mechanisms against aggression.At the cellular level, white blood cells have a role in these mechanisms with different cells with well-organized functions.

1.2 Chronic Inflammation

It is a long-term inflammation, which is often caused due to allergies, cancer, diabetes, lung diseases, asthma, heart complexities, etc. In these cases, the inflammation is cured only by treating the root cause.

Inflammation may be the defense reply that centers your immune system's consideration toward combating a perceived menace -- often microorganisms or Trojans or harm from international invaders, like poisons. When a part of your body becomes reddened, swollen, very hot and often agonizing, this is swelling in action.

Great up to now. But when swelling is chronically fired up, the immune system's capability to fight off different insects and pathogens will be compromised.

Chronic inflammation is frequently regarded as the effect of your "overactive" disease fighting capability -- as if your immune purpose is perplexed or malfunctioning. But can be this definitely what's going on? Or carry out we just reside in an increasingly harmful and stressful entire world?

After all, a lot of people today are confused with anxiety and environmental poisons, like endocrine-disrupting and cancer-causing substances from food to drinking water to household cleansers. And your body has every right to respond defensively. Foods allergies, poor diet program, toxins, and pressure are the most important culprits.

To combat irritation, we have to help our anatomies deal with this continuous harm of immune causes. One of the better ways to aid your body in combatting inflammation would be to consume an anti-inflammatory diet program.

Inflammation is a useful reaction since it constitutes a defense system of the body against aggression.In some cases, the inflammation may persist until it becomes chronic.The immune system is then overwhelmed by this inflammatory reaction.It is no longer beneficial at all and must be diagnosed and treated with medication.This is the case with chronic inflammatory diseases, such as rheumatoid arthritis or Crohn's disease.

This is why, when the inflammation becomes chronic, that is to say, that it lasts and that no obvious cause is found, it is necessary to consult your doctor to do research to find the cause of this inflammation: search for an autoimmune disease, cancer, inflammatory rheumatic or digestive disease, etc.

The inflammatory response is a complex phenomenon, which can sometimes be relieved by the use of anti-inflammatory molecules such as corticosteroids or non-steroidal anti-inflammatory drugs.However, these drugs should not be used without medical advice and cannot be prescribed for all inflammatory conditions.

1.3 Acute Inflammation

It is the instantaneous response of the body to the result of damage to body cells. Swelling occurs within 2 to 3 seconds of the injury. It doesn't persist for a longer duration.

Acute inflammation is one that starts quickly and becomes serious in a brief time. Signs or symptoms are normally just present for a couple of days and nights but may persist for a couple of weeks in some instances.

Acute inflammation is characterized by several symptoms: redness at the site of infection or injury,edema(swelling), feeling hot, and pain.If the inflammatory reaction affects an organ, the function of the organ may be affected and diminished."All organs can be affected," explains Professor Ricci.In medical terminology, the inflammation of an organ is qualified by adding the suffix "ite."For example,arthritismeans inflammation of an artery andmeningitismeans inflammation of the membrane that surrounds the brain."

CHAPTER 2: HEALTH CONDITIONS ASSOCIATED WITH INFLAMMATION

2.1 Acute Bronchitis

Is an inflammation of the bronchi, which are the air pathways between the mouth and nose as well as the lungs is known as bronchitis. With bronchitis, the lining of the bronchi becomes swollen. Persons suffering from bronchitis will have a depressed ability to breathe oxygen and air into their lungs, including the inability to clear phlegm from their airways. Bacteria, viruses or other particles can cause irritation of the bronchial tubes leading to bronchitis. In most cases, acute bronchitis is a temporary illness that follows a viral or cold infection. On the other hand, chronic bronchitis refers to long-term illness and can occur due to environmental factors as well as due to an extended illness. Smoking cigarettes is a common cause of chronic bronchitis.

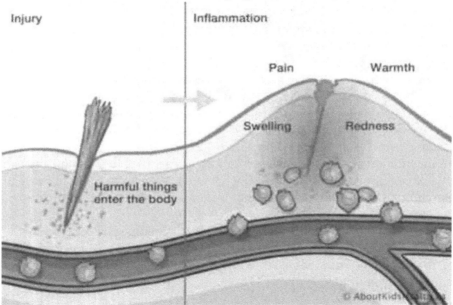

Symptoms of acute and chronic bronchitis

Wheezing

Persistent productive cough

Chest tightening

Low fever and chills

Sore throat

Breathlessness

Body aches

Headaches

Sinuses and blocked nose

2.2 Sore throat

Sore throat refers to any condition that makes the throat tender, scratchy, and painful. Strep throat is an inflammation of the throat caused by a particular strain of bacteria. The bacteria streptococcal are extremely contagious. Compared to adults, children are more vulnerable since their immune systems have had fewer encounters with germs. Medical assistance should be sought for a sore throat that causes difficulty in breathing.

Symptoms of a strep throat

Difficulty swallowing

Pain in the throat

Fever

Loss of appetite

Tonsils are inflamed thus swollen or painful

Lymph glands of the neck are swollen and tender

Small red spots may appear on the roof of the mouth

Some people may lack any signs and may not feel unwell even though they are still infectious

2.3 Acute Appendicitis

A condition where the appendix becomes inflamed, swollen, and filled with pus is known as appendicitis. The specific role of an appendix in human beings is not clear, but the area can host friendly bacteria that aid in the digestion of food and fight infection. The appendix may also be part of the immune system and impact the ability of the body to fight off infection. Appendicitis may arise mainly due to stomach infection moving to the appendix. A hard piece of stool that becomes trapped in the appendix can also cause infection.

Symptoms of appendicitis

Pain across the abdominal area is the first sign of appendicitis.

The site of the pain becomes more felt in the lower-right hand side of the abdomen as the infection progresses in an area called McBurney's point.

Gradually worsening pain

Nausea

Painful sneezing or coughing

Vomiting

Diarrhea

Fever

Inability to break wind

Constipation

Loss of appetite

Diagnosis

Almost half of the patients with appendicitis lack any telling symptoms and this makes diagnosis difficult. For instance, pain in some cases of appendicitis is not always located in the right lower quadrant of the abdomen. Other conditions may also have similar symptoms:

Urinary tract infection
Gastroenteritis
Ectopic pregnancy
Kidney stones
Crohn's disease

2.4 Dermatitis

Any inflammation of the skin is called dermatitis and can have many causes and manifest in several forms. Dermatitis is normally reddened skin, an itchy rash on the inflamed skin. Skins affected by dermatitis may ooze, blister, flake off or develop a crust. Eczema is an example of dermatitis that is atopic. Contact with poison ivy, jewelry with nickel and soaps can cause dandruff. Even though dermatitis is common, it is not contagious, but it makes you feel self-conscious and uncomfortable. Treating dermatitis requires a combination of self-care steps and medications.

Symptoms

Eczema or atopic dermatitis normally starts at infancy as a red, itchy rash that occurs where the skin flexes, such as the inside the elbows, the front of the neck, and the behind of the knees. The rash can leak fluid or crust over when scratched. Individuals with atopic dermatitis can experience relief followed by flare-ups. Eczema is caused by multiple factors such as gene variation, dry skin, environmental conditions, skin bacteria, and dysfunction of the immune system.

Contact dermatitis is a rash that occurs on sites of the body that have come into interaction with substances that cause an allergic reaction or irritate the skin. Soap, poison ivy, and essential oils can cause irritation or allergic reaction on the skin. The contact dermatitis rash may itch, burn or sting and blisters can also develop. Therefore, contact dermatitis arises from direct contact with any of the irritants or allergens, including preservatives in lotions and creams.

Seborrheic dermatitis refers to a condition that causes red skin, scaly patches, and persistent dandruff. Seborrhea dermatitis normally affects oily areas of the boy, notably the face, back, and upper chest. The condition can be a long-term condition with bouts of remission and recurrences. Seborrheic dermatitis can be caused by a fungus that is in the oil secretion on the skin. Seborrhea symptoms may come and go depending on the season.

2.5 Eczema and food

There can be food-specific eczema reactions, and they normally happen within six to twenty-four hours after eating the offending food. The reactions can also take longer than usual. A doctor will prescribe an elimination diet to help determine what foods may be triggering the reaction. An elimination diet involves cutting out certain most common foods known to trigger eczema. Prior to eliminating any food, an individual will need to carefully add each type of food into the diet and monitor eczema for four to six weeks to figure out if they are reactive to any specific food.

Consider avoiding a specific food added to the diet that worsens symptoms of eczema. If symptoms do not improve with the elimination, the specific food should not be purged from the diet as you are not reactive to it.

Common foods that can trigger or worsen eczema and should be avoided from your diet include:

Dairy

Citrus fruits

Eggs

Soy

Wheat or gluten

Cloves, cinnamon, and vanilla including other spices

Some types of nuts

Tomatoes

Some doctors may suggest allergy testing even if an individual is not allergic to a particular food and they experience sensitivity to it and can experience skin symptoms after recurrent exposure. It is called food responsive eczema reaction. Eating foods that do not contain nickel may benefit individuals with dyshidrotic eczema that tends to affect feet and hands. Soil contains a trace amount of nickel which implies that it can be present in foods.

Nickel-containing foods include:

Black tea

Beans

Canned meats

Lentils

Nuts

Chocolate

Shellfish

Peas

Soybeans

Seeds

Certain individuals with eczema also have an oral allergy syndrome or birch pollen sensitivity and may have reactions to the following foods:

Carrot

Green apples

Celery

Pears

Hazelnuts

Individuals with eczema are more susceptible to oral allergy syndrome.

2.5 Tonsillitis

An infection of the tonsils is known as tonsillitis.

Situated at the back of the throat, tonsils act as a collection site of lymphoid tissue that constitutes the immune system. Even though unpleasant and uncomfortable, tonsillitis rarely leads to major health concerns. Tonsillitis resolve on their account without any need for intervention and symptoms clear seven to ten days. Bacteria or viruses can cause a tonsil infection. A bacterial swab and examination of the throat can be used to diagnose tonsillitis.

A range of pathogens can cause tonsillitis and tonsils are the first line of defense against the external pathogen in the body.

Symptoms

High temperature

Sore throat

Pain when swallowing

Red and swollen tonsils that are pus-filled spots

Headache

Earache and pain in the neck

Coughing

Fatigue

Chills

Difficulty sleeping

Enlarged lymph glands

2.6 Sinusitis

Inflammation of the paranasal sinuses, which are the cavities that generate mucus required for the nasal passages to work effectively, is known as sinusitis. Sinusitis can be chronic or acute. Fungi, bacteria, viruses, autoimmune reactions or allergies can cause sinusitis. In most cases, sinusitis does not require medical intervention, but if symptoms last more than seven to ten days or if there is a bad headache or fever.

Symptoms

Blocked nose

Yellow or green nasal discharge that is thick

Facial pressure and pain

The depressed sense of smell

Cough

Congestion

Halitosis

Fever

Headache

Toothache

Should these symptoms persist for at least twelve weeks, then the person will be diagnosed as having chronic sinusitis.

2.7 Heart Attacks and Strokes

Scientists argue that when the inflammatory cells stay in the blood for longer than they should, it leads to a condition known as plague (Pechous et al., 2015). The plague is perceived by the immune system as a foreign invader in the body and as such, your system strives to prevent the plague within the blood vessels from getting inside arteries. Over time, the plague may become wobbly and rupture, forming a lump that blocks sufficient blood flow throughout the body. Consequently, this leads to the condition of stroke or heart attack, otherwise known as cardiovascular disease (CVD), which is among the highest cause of mortality in the developed nations.

2.8 Cancer

While the connection isn't perfectly understood, there have been studies examining the link between inflammation and cancer. What has been discovered is that inflammation can damage DNA, and these mutations are what we recognize as cancer. Inflammation can also stimulate tumor growth by producing cytokine molecules, which aid in bringing oxygen and nutrients to tumors (Danovi, 2013). Tumors are cancerous growths amassed by cancer cells, and allowing them to thrive unchecked can lead to the spread of cancer throughout the body.

2.9 Type 2 Diabetes

Diabetes is characterized by an inability to produce sufficient amounts of insulin, the chemical responsible for ensuring your blood sugar levels remain steady. Insulin also helps your body use and process sugar in order to give you the energy you need to live. Scientists have discovered that people whose blood sugar levels are unregulated by insulin have higher levels of inflammation than people who don't have insulin issues (Iwata, Ota & Duman, 2013). The implication here is that chronic inflammation affects insulin function and, therefore, can lead to Type 2 diabetes.

CHAPTER 3: THE ANTI INFLAMMATORY DIET

3.1 Anti Inflammatory Diet Pyramid

An anti-inflammatory diet is ideal for anyone dealing with inflammatory conditions. This diet doesn't isn't restrictive, and anyone can follow this diet. While getting started with this diet, you must begin by reducing your intake of all kinds of unhealthy fats. To do this, you must remove all foods rich in Omega-6 fatty oils and replace them with foods rich in Omega-3 fatty acids. The best way to follow this diet is by concentrating on all the foods you can eat, instead of worrying about all that you must no longer consume. Here is a pure food pyramid that you can use to get started with this diet. Start from the base of the pyramid and slowly make your way to the top.

Stage 1

At this stage, you need to consume the rainbow. It essentially means that you must include foods of all colors. Have plenty of anti-inflammatory vegetables. Make sure that you consume about 2-3 servings of veggies for lunch and dinner. You can have 2-3 servings of fruits, including all types of berries. It can make for a quick and easy snack.

Stage 2

You can enjoy a couple of healthy carbs but in limited amounts. The healthy carbs you can include are yams, whole grains, and plantains.

Stage 3

At this stage, you can start including a small number of nuts and seeds. You can include almonds, along with oils made from nuts and seeds such as olive oil, avocado oil, and hemp oil.

Stage 4

Now, it is time to include anti-inflammatory proteins. You can consist of naturally fatty fish like salmon, herring, mackerel, and sardines caught in the wild. Also, you can consist of tempeh, tofu, and other whole soy products.

Stage 5

It is time to include other protein-rich foods like eggs, cheeses, and deskinned poultry. However, you must add them in small quantities.

Final Stage

Kudos to you! You have made it to the top of the pyramid. At this stage, you can consume plenty of spices, green tea, dark chocolate (at least 60% cacao content) along with red wine, in limited quantities. By making a couple of dietary changes and being mindful of what you eat, you can turn your life around. If you notice that certain foods trigger any food sensitivities, then get rid of them. Pay attention to the way your body reacts to the foods you consume, and you will be fine. Your body knows what it needs, so listen to it.

3.2 The Anti Inflammatory Foods

If you already eat a fairly healthy diet, you will have no trouble incorporating these foods into your meals. In fact, you may already be enjoying them and just need a few tweaks to increase their presence in your meal planning. Some of the good foods that prevent and reduce chronic inflammation are as follows:

Omega 3 Fatty Acids

Omega 3 fatty acids are found in fish and fish oil. They calm the white blood cells and help them realize there is no danger, so they will return to dormancy. Wild salmon and other fish are good sources; I recommend eating them at least three times a week. Other foods rich in Omega 3s are flax meal and dry beans such as navy beans, kidney beans, and soybeans. An Omega3 supplement may be helpful if you are not able to ingest enough of these foods.

Fruits And Vegetables

Most fruits and vegetables are anti-inflammatory. They are naturally rich in antioxidants, carotenoids, lycopene, and magnesium. Dark green leafy vegetables and colorful fruits and berries do much to inhibit white blood cell activity.

At least nine servings of fruits and vegetables each day are recommended. One serving is about a half-cup of cooked fruits and vegetables or a full cup if raw. The Mediterranean Diet, rich in fruits and vegetables, is often suggested to individuals suffering from chronic inflammation.

Protective Oils And Fats

Yes, there are a few oils and fats that are actually good for chronic inflammation sufferers. They include coconut oil and extra virgin olive oil. Butter or cream is also fine to consume. Ghee, made from butter, is even better because it has the lactose and casein removed – the very ingredients that cause so much trouble if you have lactose intolerance or wheat sensitivity.

Fiber

Fiber keeps waste moving through the body. Since the vast majority of our immune cells reside in the intestines, it is important to keep your gut happy. Eat at least 25 grams of fiber every day in the form of fresh vegetables, fruits, and whole grains. If that doesn't provide enough fiber, feel free to take a fiber supplement.

Miscellaneous

Flavor your food with spices and herbs instead of bad fats and unsafe oils. Spices like turmeric, cumin, cloves, ginger, and cinnamon can enhance the calming of white blood cells. Herbs like fennel, rosemary, sage, and thyme also aid in reducing inflammation while adding delicious new flavors to your food.

Fermented foods like sauerkraut, buttermilk, yogurt, and kimchi contain helpful bacteria that tend to prevent inflammation.

Healthy snacks would include a limited amount of unsweetened, plain yogurt with fruit mixed in, celery, carrots, pistachios, almonds, walnuts, and other fruits and vegetables.

3.3 The Inflammatory Food To Avoid On The Diet

While there are many foods that should be included in your diet to aid in reducing chronic inflammation, there are also some foods that you must avoid to help keep the inflammation down.

Processed foods and sugars are two of the biggest culprits when it comes to inflammation in the western diet. Processed foods are highly refined, causing them to lose much of their natural fiber and nutrients. They also are often high in omega 6, trans fats, and saturated fats, which all increase inflammation.

Sugar is one of the worst offenders when it comes to increased inflammation. Not only does it hide in many foods, studies have found that it is also very addictive. Because of this, you should expect to go through a withdrawal phase when you remove it from your diet. This can often cause headaches, cravings, and sluggishness. Give yourself some time to allow your body to work through it. Sugar, even natural sugars such as honey and agave, cause the body to release cytokines, which causes an immune response leading to inflammation. You don't have to fully remove natural sugars from your diet, but you should work towards only eating them a few times a week and at no more than one meal per day.

Most fried foods, especially deep-fried foods, should be avoided as well. Usually, they are cooked in processed oils or lard and are coated in a refined flour that promotes inflammation.

You will want to pay attention to foods known as nightshades. Nightshades can be anti-inflammatory, but some people are sensitive to them, if you find you seem to have more inflammation after consuming nightshade, you may want to begin to make substitutions in your recipes.

3.4 Specific Guide On What To Eat And What To Avoid

Next page are many of the foods to increase in your diet as well as ones you should limit or avoid. This list is not all-inclusive, so remember to stick to the above points.

Foods to Enjoy	Foods to Avoid
Vegetables Kale String Beans Spinach Water Chestnut Collards Cauliflower Arugula Fennel Broccoli Lettuce Carrots Peppers Cabbage Rhubarb Artichoke Shallots AsparagusMushrooms Beets Garlic Brussel SproutsOnion ZucchiniLeeks Squash Radishes WatercressChard	**Vegetables** Nightshades such as Banana Peppers Chili Peppers Thai Peppers Tomatoes Tomatillos Pimentos Sweet Peppers Habanero Eggplant Jalapeno Potatoes (sweet potatoes are ok)

BeetsBok Choy Celery Cucumber Turnips **Fruits** Apple Blueberries WatermelonPomegranate Apricot Cantaloupe BananaPlum StrawberriesPineapple Blackberries Cherries StarfruitPear Dates Papaya Figs Orange NectarineGrapes MangoGuava Lemon Honeydew Kiwi Clementine	Artichoke All canned and frozen vegetables should be avoided. **Fruits** All canned and frozen fruits should be avoided.
Vegetarian Protein Tempeh Soy Nuts Edamame Soy Milk Tofu Organic Eggs	**Vegetarian Protein** Dairy Frozen or processed meals Nonorganic eggs
Protein TunaFlounder Clams Shrimp Striped Bass Rainbow Trout SnapperSardines Crab Halibut Herring Salmon Lobster Oysters Skinless ChickenOrganic Eggs	**Protein** Red meat with hormones Processed meats such as deli meat, hot dogs, bacon, and sausage.
Grains Barley Black Rice Wild Rice Quinoa Brown Rice Oats Buckwheat Millet Bulgar Farro Corn	**Grains** White Rice Wheat Flour Corn
Starchy Vegetables Acorn Squash Yams Jicama Butternut Squash Gold Potatoes Parsnips Red Potatoes Artichoke Sweet Potatoes Pumpkin	**Starchy Vegetables** White Potatoes may cause inflammation for those sensitive to nightshades.

Purple Potatoes White Potatoes	
Fats and Oils Almonds Avocado Oil Almond Butter Cashews Almond Oil Cashew Butter Olive Oil Hazelnuts WalnutsChia Seeds Walnut OilSesame Seed Oil Hemp seedsFlax Seeds AvocadoBrazil Nuts Pumpkin Seeds Pecans Macadamia NutsOlives Sunflower Seed Butter	**Fats and Oils** Vegetable Oil Safflower Oil Soybean Oil Grapeseed Oil Peanut Butter Mayonnaise Corn Oil
Herbs and Spices Turmeric Garlic Ginger Cinnamon Basil Thyme Black PepperSage Cilantro Parsley Cayenne Pepper Oregano Dill Mint Cloves Cumin	**Herbs and Spices** Cayenne Pepper and Chili Pepper may cause inflammation to those sensitive to nightshades.
Beverages Water Tea-Green, Black, White, Herbal, and Oolong	**Beverages** All other beverages should be avoided.
Nightshade Substitutions White Potato- Sweet Potato, Parsnips, or Turnips. Tomatoes- Beets, Pumpkin or Butternut Squash. Bell Peppers- Carrots, Celery, Cucumbers, or Radishes. Chili and Cayenne Pepper- Turmeric, Black Pepper, Cloves, Ginger or Garlic Powder. Eggplant- Portobello Mushrooms, Zucchini, or Okra.	

CHAPTER 4: BREAKFAST AND BRUNCH

Turmeric Oven Scrambled Eggs

Preparation Time: 10 minutes

Cooking Time: 15 minutes

Servings: 6

Ingredients:

8 to 10 large eggs, pasture-raised

½ cup unsweetened almond or coconut milk

½ teaspoon turmeric powder

1 teaspoon chopped cilantro

¼ teaspoon black pepper

A pinch of salt

Directions:

Preheat the oven to 3500F.

Grease a casserole or heat-proof baking dish.

In a bowl, whisk the egg, milk, turmeric powder, black pepper and salt.

Pour in the egg mixture into the baking dish.

Place in the oven and bake for 15 minutes or until the eggs have set.

Remove from the oven and garnish with chopped cilantro on top.

Nutrition:

Calories 203

Total Fat 16g

Saturated Fat 4g

Total Carbs 5g

Net Carbs 4g

Protein 10g

Sugar: 4g

Fiber: 1g

Sodium: 303 mg

Potassium 321mg

Breakfast Oatmeal

Preparation Time: 5minutes

Cooking Time: 8 minutes

Servings: 1

Ingredients:

2/3 cup coconut milk

1 egg white, pasture-raised

½ cup gluten-free quick-cooking oats

½ teaspoon turmeric powder

½ teaspoon cinnamon

¼ teaspoon ginger

Directions:

Place the non-dairy milk in a saucepan and heat over medium flame.

Stir in the egg white and continue whisking until the mixture becomes smooth.

Add in the rest of the ingredients and cook for another 3 minutes.

Nutrition:

Calories 395

Total Fat 34g

Saturated Fat 7g

Total Carbs 19g

Net Carbs 16g

Protein 10g

Sugar: 2g

Fiber: 3g

Sodium: 76mg

Potassium 459mg

Blueberry Smoothie

Preparation Time: 5 minutes

Cooking Time: 0 minutes

Servings: 1

Ingredients:

1 cup almond milk

1 frozen banana

1 cup frozen blueberries

2 handful spinach

1 tablespoon almond butter

¼ teaspoon cinnamon

¼ teaspoon cayenne pepper

1 teaspoon maca powder

Directions:

Combine all ingredients in a blender and pulse until well-combined.

Serve immediately.

Nutrition:

Calories 431

Total Fat 21g

Saturated Fat 4g

Total Carbs 56g

Net Carbs 48g

Protein 10g

Sugar: 38g

Fiber: 8g

Sodium: 201mg

Potassium 807mg

Breakfast Porridge

Preparation Time: 15 minutes,

Cooking Time: 0 minutes;

Servings: 1

Ingredients:

6 tablespoons organic cottage cheese

3 tablespoons flaxseed

3 tablespoons flax oil

2 tablespoons organic raw almond butter

1 tablespoon organic coconut meat

1 tablespoon raw honey

¼ cup water

Directions:

Combine all ingredients in a bowl. Mix until well combined.

Place in a bowl and chill before serving.

Nutrition:

Calories 632

Total Fat 49g

Saturated Fat 5g

Total Carbs 32g

Net Carbs 26g

Protein 23g

Sugar: 22g Fiber: 6g

Sodium: 265mg Potassium 533mg

Quinoa and Asparagus Mushroom Frittata

Preparation Time: 5 minutes

Cooking Time: 30 minutes

Servings: 3

Ingredients:

2 tablespoons olive oil

1 cup sliced mushrooms

1 cup asparagus, cut into 1-inch pieces

½ cup chopped tomato

6 large eggs, pasture-raised

2 large egg whites, pasture-raised

¼ cup non-dairy milk

1 cup quinoa, cooked according to the package

3 tablespoons chopped basil

1 tablespoon chopped parsley, garnish

Salt and pepper to taste

Directions:

Preheat the oven to 3500F.

In a skillet, heat the olive oil over medium flame.

Stir in the mushrooms and asparagus.

Season with salt and pepper to taste. Sauté for 7 minutes or until the mushrooms and asparagus have browned.

Add the tomatoes and cook for another 3 minutes. Set aside.

Meanwhile, mix the eggs, egg white, and milk in a mixing bowl. Set aside.

Place in a baking dish the quinoa and top with the vegetable mixture. Pour in the egg mixture.

Place in the oven and bake for 20 minutes or until the eggs have set.

Nutrition:

Calories 450

Total Fat 37g

Saturated Fat 5g

Total Carbs 17g

Net Carbs 14g

Protein 12g

Sugar: 2g

Fiber: 3g

Sodium: 60mg

Potassium 349mg

Anti-Inflammatory Cherry Spinach Smoothie

Preparation Time: 5 minutes

Cooking Time: 0 minutes

Servings: 1

Ingredients:

1 cup plain kefir

1 cup frozen cherries, pitted

½ cup baby spinach leaves

¼ cup mashed ripe avocado

1 tablespoon almond butter

1-piece peeled ginger (1/2 inch)

1 teaspoon chia seeds

Directions:

Place all ingredients in a blender.

Pulse until smooth.

Allow to chill in the fridge before serving.

Nutrition:

Calories 410

Total Fat 20g

Saturated Fat 4g

Total Carbs 47g

Net Carbs 37g

Protein 17g

Sugar: 33g

Fiber: 10g

Sodium: 169mg

Potassium 1163mg

Tropical Carrot Ginger and Turmeric Smoothie

Preparation Time: 5 minutes

Cooking Time: 0 minutes

Servings: 1

Ingredients:

1 blood orange, peeled and seeded

1 large carrot, peeled and chopped

½ cup frozen mango chunks

2/3 cup coconut water

1 tablespoon raw hemp seeds

¾ teaspoon grated ginger

1 ½ teaspoon peeled and grated turmeric

A pinch of cayenne pepper

A pinch of salt

Directions:

Place all ingredients in a blender and blend until smooth.

Chill before serving.

Nutrition:

Calories 259

Total Fat 6g

Saturated Fat 0.9g

Total Carbs 51g

Net Carbs 40g

Protein 7g

Sugar: 34g

Fiber: 11g

Sodium: 225mg

Potassium 1319mg

Golden Milk Chia Pudding

Preparation Time: 6 hours

Cooking Time: 0 minutes

Servings: 4

Ingredients:

4 cups coconut milk

3 tablespoons honey

1 teaspoon vanilla extract

1 teaspoon ground turmeric

½ teaspoon ground cinnamon

½ teaspoon ground ginger

¾ cup coconut yogurt

½ cup chia seeds

1 cup fresh mixed berry

¼ cup toasted coconut chips

Directions:

In a mixing bowl, combine the coconut milk, honey, vanilla extract, turmeric, cinnamon, and ginger. Add in the coconut yogurt.

In bowls, place chia seeds, berries, and coconut chips.

Pour in the milk mixture.

Allow to chill in the fridge to set for 6 hours.

Nutrition:

Calories 337

Total Fat 11g

Saturated Fat 2g

Total Carbs 51g

Net Carbs 49g

Protein 10g

Sugar: 29g

Fiber: 2g

Sodium: 262mg

Potassium 508mg

No-Bake Turmeric Protein Donuts

Preparation Time: 50 minutes

Cooking Time: 0 minutes

Servings: 8

Ingredients:

1 ½ cups raw cashews

½ cup medjool dates, pitted

1 tablespoon vanilla protein powder

½ cup shredded coconut

2 tablespoons maple syrup

¼ teaspoon vanilla extract

1 teaspoon turmeric powder

¼ cup dark chocolate

Directions:

Combine all ingredients except for the chocolate in a food processor.

Pulse until smooth.

Roll batter into 8 balls and press into a silicone donut mold.

Place in the freezer for 30 minutes to set.

Meanwhile, make the chocolate topping by melting the chocolate in a double boiler. Once the donuts have set, remove the donuts from the mold and drizzle with chocolate.

Nutrition:

Calories 320

Total Fat 26g

Saturated Fat 5g

Total Carbs 20g

Net Carbs 18g

Protein 7g

Sugar: 9g

Fiber: 2g

Sodium: 163 mg

Potassium 297mg

Choco-Nana Pancakes

Preparation Time: 5 minutes

Cooking Time: 6 minutes

Servings: 2

Ingredients:

2 large bananas, peeled and mashed

2 large eggs, pasture-raised

3 tablespoon cacao powder

2 tablespoons almond butter

1 teaspoon pure vanilla extract

1/8 teaspoon salt

Coconut oil for greasing

Directions:

Preheat a skillet on medium-low heat and grease the pan with coconut oil.

Place all ingredients in a food processor and pulse until smooth.

Pour a batter (about ¼ cup) onto the skillet and form a pancake.

Cook for 3 minutes on each side.

Nutrition:

Calories 303

Total Fat 17g

Saturated Fat 4g

Total Carbs 36g

Net Carbs 29g

Protein 5g

Sugar: 15g

Fiber: 5g

Sodium: 108mg

Potassium 549mg

Sweet Potato Cranberry Breakfast bars

Preparation Time: 10 minutes

Cooking Time: 40 minutes

Servings: 8

Ingredients:

1 ½ cups sweet potato puree

2 tablespoons coconut oil, melted

2 tablespoons maple syrup

2 eggs, pasture-raised

1 cup almond meal

1/3 cup coconut flour

1 ½ teaspoon baking soda

1 cup fresh cranberry, pitted and chopped

¼ cup water

Directions:

Preheat the oven to 3500F.

Grease a 9-inch baking pan with coconut oil. Set aside.

In a mixing bowl. Combine the sweet potato puree, water, coconut oil, maple syrup, and eggs.

In another bowl, sift the almond flour, coconut flour, and baking soda.

Gradually add the dry ingredients to the wet ingredients. Use a spatula to fold and mix all ingredients.

Pour into the prepared baking pan and press the cranberries on top.

Place in the oven and bake for 40 minutes or until a toothpick inserted in the middle comes out clean.

Allow to rest or cool before removing from the pan.

Nutrition:

Calories 98

Total Fat 6g

Saturated Fat 1g

Total Carbs 9g

Net Carbs 8.5g

Protein 3g

Sugar: 7g

Fiber: 0.5g

Sodium: 113 mg

Potassium 274mg

Savory Breakfast Pancakes

Preparation Time: 5 minutes

Cooking Time: 6 minutes

Servings: 4

Ingredients:

½ cup almond flour

½ cup tapioca flour

1 cup coconut milk

½ teaspoon chili powder

¼ teaspoon turmeric powder

½ red onion, chopped

1 handful cilantro leaves, chopped

½ inch ginger, grated

1 teaspoon salt

¼ teaspoon ground black pepper

Directions:

In a mixing bowl, mix all ingredients until well-combined.

Heat a pan on low medium heat and grease with oil.

Pour ¼ cup of batter onto the pan and spread the mixture to create a pancake.

Fry for 3 minutes per side.

Repeat until the batter is done.

Nutrition:

Calories 108

Total Fat 2g

Saturated Fat 1g

Total Carbs 20g

Net Carbs 19.5g

Protein 2g

Sugar: 4g

Fiber: 0.5g

Sodium: 37mg

Potassium 95mg

Scrambled Eggs with Smoked Salmon

Preparation Time: 10 minutes

Cooking Time: 10 minutes

Servings: 2

Ingredients:

4 eggs

2 tablespoons coconut milk

Fresh chives, chopped

4 slices of wild-caught smoked salmon, chopped

Salt to taste

Directions:

In a bowl, whisk the egg, coconut milk, and chives.

Grease the skillet with oil and heat over medium-low heat.

Pour the egg mixture and scramble the eggs while cooking.

When the eggs start to settle, add in the smoked salmon and cook for 2 more minutes.

Nutrition:

Calories 349

Total Fat 23g

Saturated Fat 4g

Total Carbs 3g

Net Carbs 1g

Protein 29g

Sugar: 2g

Fiber: 2g

Sodium: 466mg

Potassium 536mg

Raspberry Grapefruit Smoothie

Preparation Time: 5 minutes

Cooking Time: 0 minutes

Servings: 1

Ingredients:

Juice from 1 grapefruit, freshly squeezed

1 banana, peeled and sliced

1 cup raspberries

Directions:

Place all ingredients in a blender and pulse until smooth.

Chill before serving.

Nutrition:

Calories 381

Total Fat 0.8g

Saturated Fat 0.1g

Total Carbs 96g

Net Carbs 85g

Protein 4g

Sugar: 61g

Fiber: 11g

Sodium: 11mg

Potassium 848mg

Breakfast Burgers with Avocado Buns

Preparation Time: 10 minutes

Cooking Time: 5 minutes

Servings: 1

Ingredients:

1 ripe avocado

1 egg, pasture-raised

1 red onion slice

1 tomato slice

1 lettuce leaf

Sesame seed for garnish

Salt to taste

Directions:

Peel the avocado and remove the seed. Slice the avocado into half. This will serve as the bun. Set aside.

Grease a skillet over medium flame and fry the egg's sunny side up for 5 minutes or until set.

Assemble the breakfast burger by placing on top of one avocado half with the egg, red onion, tomato, and lettuce leaf.

Top with the remaining avocado bun.

Garnish with sesame seeds on top and season with salt to taste.

Nutrition:

Calories 458

Total Fat 39g

Saturated Fat 4g

Total Carbs 20g

Net Carbs 6g,

Protein 13g

Sugar: 8g

Fiber: 14g

Sodium: 118mg

Potassium 1184mg

Buckwheat and Chia Seed Porridge

Preparation Time: 10 minutes

Cooking Time: 20 minutes

Servings: 5

Ingredients:

Chia Seeds 2 tablespoons

Water 2 cups

1 Apple

1 Pear

Oats 0.5 cups

Buckwheat 1 cup (rinsed)

A pinch of Ginger

Cinnamon

Cardamom

Nutmeg

Nut butter 2 tablespoons

Vanilla Extract 1 teaspoon

Honey 2 tablespoons.

Directions

Put 1 cup of milk in a bowl and add the chia seeds.

Put 1 cup of water in another bowl and add the buckwheat and oats

Leave both bowls to soak overnight

In the morning, drain water from both buckwheat and oats, rinsing them thoroughly

Place a medium saucepan over medium heat

Place the chia seeds with the milk into the saucepan.

Add the remaining milk (1 cup). Also add the other ingredients (nut butter, grated apple and pear, vanilla, honey, buckwheat, oats, and all of the spices)

Simmer and cook for 18 minutes, constantly stirring to achieve a thick and creamy porridge.

As you stir, add more water to achieve the consistency you want.

Serve the porridge in cups

Nutrition:

Calories 320

Carbs 66g

Fats 3g

Protein 12g

CHAPTER 5: LUNCH

Green Soup

Preparation Time: 10 Minutes

Cooking Time: 5 Minutes

Servings: 2

Ingredients:

1 cup Water

1 cup Spinach, fresh & packed

½ of 1 Lemon, peeled

1 Zucchini, small & chopped

2 tbsp. Parsley, fresh & chopped

1 Celery Stalk, chopped

Sea Salt & Black Pepper, as needed

½ of 1 Avocado, ripe

¼ cup Basil

2 tbsp. Chia Seeds

1 Garlic clove, minced

Directions:

To make this easy blended soup, place all the ingredients in a high-speed blender and blend for 3 minutes or until smooth.

Next, you can serve it cold, or you can warm it up on low heat for a few minutes.

Nutrition:

Calories: 250Kcal

Proteins: 6.9g

Carbohydrates: 18.4g

Fat: 18.1g

Buckwheat Noodle Soup

Preparation Time: 10 Minutes

Cooking Time: 25 Minutes

Servings: 4

Ingredients:

2 cups Bok Choy, chopped

3 tbsp. Tamari

3 bundles of Buckwheat Noodles

2 cups Edamame Beans

7 oz. Shiitake Mushrooms, chopped

4 cups Water

1 tsp. Ginger, grated

Dash of Salt

1 Garlic Clove, grated

Directions:

First, place water, ginger, soy sauce, and garlic in a medium-sized pot over medium heat.

Bring the ginger-soy sauce mixture to a boil and then stir in the edamame and shiitake to it.

Continue cooking for further 7 minutes or until tender.

Next, cook the soba noodles by following the **Directions:** given in the packet until cooked. Wash and drain well.

Now, add the bok choy to shiitake mixture and cook for further one minute or until the bok choy is wilted.

Finally, divide the soba noodles among the serving bowls and top it with the mushroom mixture.

Nutrition:

Calories: 234Kcal

Proteins: 14.2g

Carbohydrates: 35.1g

Fat: 4g

Zoodles

Preparation Time: 10 Minutes

Cooking Time: 25 Minutes

Servings: 2

Ingredients:

2 tsp. Lemon Juice

2 Zucchini, small & spiralized

1 cup Basil, fresh

8 Cherry Tomatoes

2 tbsp. Walnuts, chopped

2 tbsp. Nutritional Yeast

¼ cup Green Olives

3 Sun-dried Tomatoes, soaked

Salt & Pepper, to taste

Directions:

For making this healthy fare, you need to make zoodles out of zucchini by using a spiralizer.

After that, season the zoodles with salt and set it aside.

Then, blend all the ingredients, excluding the cherry tomatoes and olives, in a high-speed blender and blend until smooth.

Next, stir in the tomatoes and olives to it and pulse again. Tip: There should be some chunks in it.

Now, chop the walnuts and nutritional yeast in a small blender until combined well.

Finally, mix the zoodles with the pesto and then top it with the walnuts yeast mixture.

Nutrition:

Calories: 224Kcal

Proteins: 15.2g

Carbohydrates: 32.4g

Fat: 7.5g

Chickpea Curry

Preparation Time: 10 Minutes

Cooking Time: 25 Minutes

Servings: 4 to 6

Ingredients:

2 × 15 oz. Chickpeas, washed, drained & cooked

2 tbsp. Olive Oil

1 tbsp. Turmeric Powder

½ of 1 Onion, diced

1 tsp. Cayenne, grounded

4 Garlic cloves, minced

2 tsp. Chili Powder

15 oz. Tomato Puree

Black Pepper, as needed

2 tbsp. Tomato Paste

1 tsp. Cayenne, grounded

½ tbsp. Maple Syrup

½ of 15 oz. can of Coconut Milk

2 tsp. Cumin, grounded

2 tsp. Smoked Paprika

Directions:

Heat a large skillet over medium-high heat. To this, spoon in the oil.

Once the oil becomes hot, stir in the onion and cook for 3 to 4 minutes or until softened.

Next, spoon in the tomato paste, maple syrup, all seasonings, tomato puree, and garlic into it. Mix well.

Then, add the cooked chickpeas to it along with coconut milk, black pepper, and salt.

Now, give everything a good stir and allow it to simmer for 8 to 10 minutes or until thickened.

Drizzle lime juice over it and garnish with cilantro, if desired.

Nutrition:

Calories: 224Kcal

Proteins: 15.2g

Carbohydrates: 32.4g

Fat: 7.5g

Ratatouille

Preparation Time: 10 Minutes

Cooking Time: 25 Minutes

Servings: 8

Ingredients:

1 Zucchini, medium & diced

3 tbsp. Extra Virgin Olive Oil

2 Bell Pepper, diced

1 Yellow Squash, medium & diced

1 Onion, large & diced

28 oz. Whole Tomatoes, peeled

1 Eggplant, medium & diced with skin on

Salt & Pepper, as needed

4 Thyme Sprigs, fresh

5 Garlic cloves, chopped

Directions:

To start with, heat a large sauté pan over medium-high heat.

Once hot, spoon in the oil, onion, and garlic to it.

Sauté the onion mixture for 3 to 5 minutes or until softened.

Next, stir in the eggplant, pepper, thyme, and salt to the pan. Mix well.

Now, cook for further 5 minutes or until the eggplant becomes softened.

Then, add zucchini, bell peppers, and squash to the pan and continue cooking for another 5 minutes. Then, stir in the tomatoes and mix well.

Once everything is added, give a good stir until everything comes together. Allow it to simmer for 15 minutes.

Finally, check for seasoning and spoon in more salt and pepper if needed.

Garnish with parsley and ground black pepper.

Nutrition:

Calories: 103Kcal

Proteins: 2g

Carbohydrates: 12g

Fat: 5g

Herbed Baked Salmon

Preparation Time: 10 Minutes

Cooking Time: 15 Minutes

Servings: 2

Ingredients:

10 oz. Salmon Fillet

1 tsp. Olive Oil

1 tsp. Honey

1 tsp. Tarragon, fresh

1/8 tsp. Salt

2 tsp. Dijon Mustard

¼ tsp. Thyme, dried

¼ tsp. Oregano, dried

Directions:

Preheat the oven to 425 ° F.

After that, combine all the ingredients, excluding the salmon in a medium-sized bowl.

Now, spoon this mixture evenly over the salmon.

Then, place the salmon with the skin side down on the parchment paper-lined baking sheet.

Finally, bake for 8 minutes or until the fish flakes.

Nutrition:

Calories: 239Kcal

Proteins: 31g

Carbohydrates: 3g

Fat: 11g

Carrot Soup

Preparation Time: 10 Minutes

Cooking Time: 40 Minutes

Servings: 4

Ingredients:

1 cup Butternut Squash, chopped

1 tbsp. Olive Oil

1 tbsp. Turmeric Powder

14 ½ oz. Coconut Milk, light

3 cups Carrot, chopped

1 Leek, rinsed & sliced

1 tbsp. Ginger, grated

3 cups Vegetable Broth

1 cup Fennel, chopped

Salt & Pepper, to taste

2 cloves of Garlic, minced

Directions:

Start by heating a Dutch oven over medium-high heat.

To this, spoon in the oil and then stir in fennel, squash, carrots, and leek. Mix well.

Now, sauté it for 4 to 5 minutes or until softened.

Next, add turmeric, ginger, pepper, and garlic to it. Cook for another 1 to 2 minutes.

Then, pour the broth and coconut milk to it. Combine well.

After that, bring the mixture to a boil and cover the Dutch oven.

Allow it to simmer for 20 minutes.

Once cooked, transfer the mixture to a high-speed blender and blend for 1 to 2 minutes or until you get a creamy smooth soup.

Check for seasoning and spoon in more salt and pepper if needed.

Nutrition:

Calories: 210.4Kcal

Proteins: 2.11g

Carbohydrates: 25.64g

Fat: 10.91g

Lentil Soup

Preparation Time: 10 Minutes

Cooking Time: 30 Minutes

Servings: 2

Ingredients:

2 Carrots, medium & diced

2 tbsp. Lemon Juice, fresh

1 tbsp. Turmeric Powder

1/3 cup Lentils, cooked

1 tbsp. Almonds, chopped

1 Celery Stalk, diced

1 bunch of Parsley, chopped freshly

1 Yellow Onion, large & chopped

Black Pepper, freshly grounded

1 Parsnip, medium & chopped

½ tsp. Cumin Powder

3 ½ cups Water

½ tsp. Pink Himalayan Salt

4 kale leaves, chopped roughly

Directions:

To start with, place carrots, parsnip, one tablespoon of water and onion in a medium-sized pot over medium heat.

Cook the vegetable mixture for 5 minutes while stirring it occasionally.

Next, stir in the lentils and spices into it. Combine well.

After that, pour water to the pot and bring the mixture to a boil.

Now, reduce the heat to low and allow it to simmer for 20 minutes.

Off the heat and remove it from the stove.

Add the kale, lemon juice, parsley, and salt to it.

Then, give a good stir until everything comes together.

Top it with almonds and serve it hot.

Nutrition:

Calories: 242Kcal

Proteins: 10g

Carbohydrates: 46g

Fat: 4g

¼ cup Miso

¼ tsp. Pepper, grounded

2 Limes

2 ½ lb. Salmon, skin-on

Dash of Cayenne Pepper

2 tbsp. Extra Virgin Olive Oil

¼ cup Miso

Directions:

First, mix the lime juice and lemon juice in a small bowl until combined well.

Next, spoon in the miso, cayenne pepper, maple syrup, olive oil, and pepper to it. Combine well.

Then, place the salmon on a parchment paper-lined baking sheet with the skin side down.

Brush the salmon generously with the miso lemon mixture.

Now, place the halved lemon and lime pieces on the sides with the cut side up.

Finally, bake them for 8 to 12 minutes or until the fish flakes.

Nutrition:

Calories: 230Kcal

Proteins: 28.3g

Carbohydrates: 6.7g

Fat: 8.7g

Miso Broiled Salmon

Preparation Time: 10 Minutes

Cooking Time: 20 Minutes

Servings: 2

Ingredients:

2 tbsp. Maple Syrup

2 Lemons

Broccoli Cauliflower Salad

Preparation Time: 10 Minutes

Cooking Time: 20 Minutes

Servings: 6

Ingredients:

¼ tsp. Black Pepper, grounded

3 cups Cauliflower Florets

1 tbsp. Vinegar

1 tsp. Honey

8 cups Kale, chopped

3 cups Broccoli Florets

4 tbsp. Extra Virgin Olive Oil

½ tsp. Salt

1 ½ tsp. Dijon Mustard

1 tsp. Honey

½ cup Cherries, dried

1/3 cup Pecans, chopped

1 cup Manchego cheese, shaved

Directions:

Preheat the oven to 450 ˚ F and place a baking sheet in the middle rack.

After that, place cauliflower and broccoli florets in a large bowl.

To this, spoon in half of the salt, two tablespoons of the oil and pepper. Toss well.

Now, transfer the mixture to the preheated sheet and bake it for 12 minutes while flipping it once in between.

Once it becomes tender and golden in color, remove it from the oven and allow it to cool completely.

In the meantime, mix the remaining two tablespoons of oil, vinegar, honey, mustard, and salt in another bowl.

Brush this mixture over the kale leaves by messaging the leaves with your hands. Set it aside for 3 to 5 minutes.

Finally, stir in the roasted vegetables, cheese, cherries, and pecan to the broccoli-cauliflower salad.

Nutrition:

Calories: 259Kcal

Proteins: 8.4g

Carbohydrates: 23.2g

Fat: 16.3g

Spinach Salad with Beans

Preparation Time: 10 Minutes

Cooking Time: 30 Minutes

Servings: 4

Ingredients:

3 tbsp. Cider Vinegar

1 Sweet Potato, peeled & diced

½ cup Basil leaves, fresh & chopped

5 tbsp. Extra Virgin Olive Oil, divided

1 tbsp. Shallot, finely sliced

½ tsp. Pepper, grounded

2 tsp. Mustard, whole-grain

¼ tsp. Salt

15 oz. Cannellini Beans, drained & washed

1 cup Red Bell Pepper, chopped

10 cups Baby Spinach

2 cups Cabbage, shredded

1/3 cup Pecans, chopped

Directions:

For making this healthy salad, you first need to preheat the oven to 425 ˚ F.

Next, place the sweet potatoes, salt, one tablespoon oil, and pepper in a large mixing bowl.

After that, transfer the mixture to a parchment paper-lined baking sheet and roast it for 10 to 15 minutes or until tender. Set it aside to cool.

Meanwhile, mix all the remaining ingredients into a food processor and process it for 5 to 1o minutes or until smooth.

Finally, mix the spinach, sweet potatoes, the remaining oil, mustard, vinegar, bell pepper, beans to the large bow. Mix everything and enjoy it.

Nutrition:

Calories: 415Kcal

Proteins: 11.8g

Carbohydrates: 44.3g

Fat: 23.6g

Goat Cheese & Bell Pepper Salad

Preparation Time: 10 Minutes

Cooking Time: 20 Minutes

Servings: 4

Ingredients:

2 tbsp. Lemon Juice, fresh

1 ½ Red Bell Pepper, large

¾ cup Goat Cheese, crumbled

2 tbsp. Extra Virgin Olive Oil

1/3 cup Red Onion, chopped

1 tbsp. Oregano, fresh & chopped

1 ½ cup Celery, diced

4 cups Spinach leaves, chopped coarsely

Directions:

First, mix oregano, oil, and lime juice in a small bowl with a whisker until combined well.

Next, check for seasoning and spoon in more salt and pepper as needed.

Then, stir in the spinach, goat cheese, bell pepper, red onion, and celery in a large bowl. To this, stir in the dressing and toss well.

Serve immediately and enjoy it.

Nutrition:

Calories: 155Kcal

Proteins: 5.7g

Carbohydrates: 8.8g

Fat: 11.5g

CHAPTER 6: SNACKS

Chickpeas and Pepper Hummus

Preparation Time: 10 minutes

Cooking Time: 0 minute

Servings: 4

Ingredients:

14 ounces canned chickpeas, no-salt-added, drained and rinsed

1 tablespoon sesame paste

2 roasted red peppers, chopped

Juice of ½ lemon

4 walnuts, chopped

Directions:

In your blender, combine the chickpeas with all the sesame paste, red peppers, lemon juice and walnuts, pulse well, divide into bowls and serve.

Nutrition:

Calories: 231

Fat: 12g

Fiber: 6g

Carbs: 15g

Protein: 14g

Lemony Chickpeas Dip

Preparation Time: 10 minutes

Cooking Time: 0 minute

Servings: 4

Ingredients:

14 ounces canned chickpeas, drained, no-salt-added, and rinsed

Zest of merely one lemon, grated

Juice of a single lemon

1 tablespoon olive oil

4 tablespoons pine nuts

½ cup coriander, chopped

Directions:

In a blender, combine the chickpeas with lemon zest, freshly squeezed lemon juice, coriander and oil, pulse well, divide into small bowls, sprinkle pine nuts at the pinnacle and serve as a conference dip.

Nutrition:

Calories: 200

Fat: 12g

Fiber: 4g

Carbs: 9g

Protein: 7g

Chili Nuts

Preparation Time: 10 minutes

Cooking Time: 10 minutes

Servings: 4

Ingredients:

½ teaspoon chili flakes

1 egg white

½ teaspoon curry powder

½ teaspoon ginger powder

4 tablespoons coconut sugar

A pinch of cayenne

14 ounces mixed nuts

Directions:

In a bowl, combine the egg white with all the chili flakes, curry powder, curry powder, ginger powder, coconut sugar and cayenne and whisk well.

Add the nuts, toss well, spread them having a lined baking sheet, introduce within the oven and bake at 400 degrees F for ten mins.

Divide the nuts into bowls and serve as a snack.

Nutrition:

Calories: 234

Fat: 12g

Fiber: 5g

Carbs: 14g

Protein: 7g

Protein Bars

Preparation Time: 10 minutes

Cooking Time: 0 minute

Servings: 4

Ingredients:

4 ounces apricots, dried

2 ounces water

2 tablespoons rolled oats

1 tablespoon sunflower seeds

2 tablespoons coconut, shredded

1 tablespoon sesame seeds

1 tablespoon cranberries

3 tablespoons hemp seeds

1 tablespoon chia seeds

Directions:

In your food processor, combine the apricots while using water along with all the oats, pulse well, transfer for your bowl, add coconut, sunflower seeds, sesame seeds, cranberries, hemp and chia seeds and stir prior to getting a paste.

Roll this inside a log, wrap, cool inside fridge, slice and serve as a snack.

Nutrition:

Calories: 100

Fat: 3g

Fiber: 4g

Carbs: 8g

Protein: 5g

Red Pepper Muffins

Preparation Time: 10 minutes

Cooking Time: ½ hour

Servings: 12

Ingredients:

1 and ¾ cups whole wheat grains flour

2 teaspoons baking powder

2 tablespoons coconut sugar

A pinch of black pepper

1 egg

¾ cup almond milk

2/3 cup roasted red pepper, chopped

½ cup low-Fat: mozzarella, shredded

Directions:

In a bowl, combine the flour with baking powder, coconut sugar, black pepper, egg, milk, red pepper and mozzarella.

Stir well and divide in a very lined muffin tray.

Put in the oven and bake at 400 degrees F for a half-hour.

Serve like a snack.

Nutrition:

Calories: 149

Fat: 4g

Fiber: 2g

Carbs: 14g

Protein: 5g

Nuts and Seeds Mix

Preparation Time: 10 minutes

Cooking Time: 0 minutes

Servings: 6

Ingredients:

1 cup pecans

1 cup hazelnuts

1 cup almonds

¼ cup coconut, shredded

1 cup walnuts

½ cup papaya pieces, dried

½ cup dates, dried, pitted and chopped

½ cup sunflower seeds

½ cup pumpkin seeds

1 cup raisins

Directions:

In a bowl, combine the pecans with all the hazelnuts, almonds, coconut, walnuts, papaya, dates, sunflower seeds, pumpkin seeds and raisins.

Toss and serve as a snack.

Nutrition:

Calories: 188

Fat: 4g

Fiber: 6g

Carbs: 8g

Protein: 6g

Tortilla Chips

Preparation Time: 10 minutes

Cooking Time: 25 minutes

Servings: 6

Ingredients:

12 whole wheat grains tortillas, cut into 6 wedges each

2 tablespoons organic extra virgin olive oil

1 tablespoon chili powder

A pinch of cayenne

Directions:

Spread the tortillas for the lined baking sheet, add the oil, chili powder and cayenne.

Toss and put inside the oven and bake at 350 degrees F for 25 minutes.

Divide into bowls and serve as a side dish.

Nutrition:

Calories: 199

Fat: 3g

Fiber: 4g

Carbs: 12g

Protein: 5g

Kale Chips

Preparation Time: 10 minutes

Cooking Time: 15 minutes

Servings: 8

Ingredients:

1 bunch kale leaves

1 tablespoon organic olive oil

1 teaspoon smoked paprika

A pinch of black pepper

Directions:

Spread the kale leaves over a baking sheet, add black pepper, oil and paprika.

Toss and put inside the oven and bake at 350 degrees F for quarter-hour.

Divide into bowls and serve being a snack.

Nutrition:

Calories: 177

Fat: 2g

Fiber: 4g

Carbs: 13g

Protein: 6g

Potato Chips

Preparation Time: 10 minutes

Cooking Time: 30 minutes

Servings: 6

Ingredients:

2 gold potatoes, cut into thin rounds

1 tablespoon olive oil

2 teaspoons garlic, minced

Directions:

In a bowl, combine the French fries while using the oil along with the garlic, toss, spread more than a lined baking sheet.

Put inside the oven and bake at 400 degrees F for a half-hour.

Divide into bowls and serve.

Nutrition:

Calories: 200,

Fat: 3,

Fiber: 5,

Carbs: 13,

Protein: 6

Peach Dip

Preparation Time: 10 minutes

Cooking Time: 0 minute

Servings: 2

Ingredients:

½ cup nonfat: yogurt

1 cup peaches, chopped

A pinch of cinnamon powder

A pinch of nutmeg, ground

Directions:

In a bowl, combine the yogurt while using the peaches, cinnamon and nutmeg.

Whisk and divide into small bowls and serve.

Nutrition:

Calories: 165

Fat: 2g

Fiber: 3g

Carbs: 14g

Protein: 13g

Cereal Mix

Preparation Time: 10 minutes

Cooking Time: 40 minutes

Servings: 6

Ingredients:

3 tablespoons extra virgin organic olive oil

1 teaspoon hot sauce

½ teaspoon garlic powder

½ teaspoon onion powder

½ teaspoon cumin, ground

A pinch of red pepper cayenne

3 cups rice cereal squares

1 cup cornflakes

½ cup pepitas

Directions:

In a bowl, combine the oil while using the hot sauce, garlic powder, onion powder, cumin, cayenne, rice cereal, cornflakes and pepitas.

Toss and spread on the lined baking sheet.

Put inside the oven and bake at 350 degrees F for 40 minutes.

Divide into bowls and serve as a snack.

Nutrition:

Calories: 199

Fat: 3g

Fiber: 4g

Carbs: 12g Protein: 5g

Eggplant, Olives and Basil Salad

Preparation Time: 15 minutes

Cooking Time: 10 minutes

Servings: 4

Ingredients:

Tomatoes, chopped: 1 ½ cups

Eggplant, cubed: 3 cups

Capers: 2 teaspoons

Green olives, pitted and sliced: 6 ounces

Minced garlic: 2 teaspoons

Salt: ½ teaspoon

Ground black pepper: ¼ teaspoon

Chopped basil: 1 tablespoon

Olive oil: 2 teaspoons

Balsamic vinegar: 2 teaspoons

Directions:

Place a medium skillet pan over medium-high heat, add oil and when hot, add eggplant pieces and cook for 5 minutes.

Then add remaining ingredients, stir well and cook for 5 minutes.

When done, remove the pan from heat and let cool for 5 minutes.

Then divide salad evenly between small cups and serve as an appetizer.

Nutrition:

Calories: 199

Fat: 6g Fiber: 5g Carbs: 7g Protein: 7g

Fresh Tomato, Onion and Jalapeno Pepper Salsa

Preparation Time: 5 minutes

Cooking Time: 0 minute

Servings: 4

Ingredients:

Cherry tomatoes, halved: 2 cups

Red onion, peeled and chopped: ¼ cup

Jalapeno pepper, chopped: 1

Minced garlic: ½ teaspoon

Chopped cilantro: 2 tablespoons

Salt: ¼ teaspoon

Ground black pepper: ¼ teaspoon

Lime juice: 2 tablespoons

Directions:

Place all the ingredients for salsa in a medium bowl and stir until combined.

Serve straight away as a snack.

Nutrition:

Calories: 87

Fat: 1g

Fiber: 2g

Carbs: 7g

Protein: 5g

Fresh Veggie Bars

Preparation Time: 40 minutes

Cooking Time: 25 minutes

Servings: 18

Ingredients:

Egg-1

Broccoli florets-2 cups

Cheddar cheese-1/3 cup (grated)

Onion-¼ cup (peeled and chopped)

Cauliflower rice-½ cup

Fresh parsley-2 tablespoons (chopped)

Olive oil-A drizzle (for greasing)

Salt and black pepper-to taste (ground)

Directions:

Warm-up a saucepan with water over medium heat

Stir into the broccoli and let it simmer for a minute.

Strain and finely chop it to put it into a bowl.

Mix in the egg, cheddar cheese, cauliflower rice, salt, pepper, parsley, and mix.

Give them the shape of bars by using the mixture on your hands.

Put them on a greased baking sheet.

Keep it in an oven at 400ºF and bake for 20 minutes.

Settle the prepared dish on a platter to serve.

Nutrition:

Calories: 19

Fat: 1g Fiber: 3g

Carbs: 3g

Protein: 3g

Green Beans and Avocado with Chopped Cilantro

Preparation Time: 15 minutes

Cooking Time: 10 minutes

Servings: 4

Ingredients:

Avocados: 2; pitted and peeled

Green beans - 2/3 pound, trimmed

Scallions - 5, chopped.

Olive oil - 3 tablespoons

A handful cilantro, chopped.

Salt and black pepper to the taste.

Directions:

Heat up a pan containing oil on a medium-high heat source; then add green beans and stir gently. Cook this mixture for about 4 minutes

Add salt and pepper to the pan, and stir gently, then remove the heat and move to a clean bowl.

Mix the avocados with salt and pepper and mash with a fork inside a clean bowl.

Then add onions and stir properly.

Add this over green beans, then toss to ensure it is well coated.

Finally, serve with some chopped cilantro on top.

Nutrition:

Calories: 200

Fat: 5g

Fiber: 3g

Carbs: 4g

Protein: 6g

Parsnip Fries

Preparation Time: 10 minutes

Cooking Time: 40 minutes

Servings: 4

Ingredients:

2 tablespoons extra-virgin olive oil

1¼ pound small parsnips, peeled and quartered

1½ tablespoons fresh ginger, minced

¼ teaspoon ground cumin

1/8 teaspoon ground turmeric

Salt and black pepper, to taste

Directions:

Adjust your oven to 325 degrees F.

In a 13x9-inch baking dish, place the oil evenly.

Add remaining ingredients and toss to coat well.

With a foil paper, cover the baking dish and bake for about 40 minutes.

Serve immediately.

Nutrition:

Calories 248

Total Fat 15.7 g

Saturated Fat 2.7 g

Cholesterol 75 mg

Sodium 94 mg

Total Carbs 15.4 g

Fiber 0g Sugar 0 g Protein 4.9 g

Spinach Chips

Preparation Time: 10 minutes

Cooking Time: 8 minutes

Total time: 18 minutes

Servings: 2

Ingredients:

2 cups fresh spinach leaves

¼ teaspoon extra-virgin olive oil

Salt, to taste

Italian seasoning, to taste

Directions:

Adjust your oven to 325 degrees F. Line a baking sheet with a parchment paper.

In a large bowl, add spinach leaves and drizzle with oil.

With your hands, rub the spinach leaves till all the leaves are coated with oil.

Transfer the leaves into the prepared baking sheet in a single layer.

Bake for about 8 minutes.

Serve immediately.

Nutrition:

Calories 287

Total Fat 29.5 g

Saturated Fat 3 g

Cholesterol 0 mg

Total Carbs 15.9 g

Sugar 1.4g

Fiber 4.3 g Sodium 388 mg

Protein 4.2 g

Fruit Salsa

Preparation Time: 10 minutes

Cooking Time: 0 minutes

Servings: 4

Ingredients:

2 cups fresh pineapple, chopped

2 mangoes, peeled, pitted and chopped

½ cup red onion, chopped

¼ cup fresh cilantro leaves, chopped

1 tablespoon fresh ginger, chopped finely

1 teaspoon red pepper flakes, crushed

¼ cup apple cider vinegar

Directions:

In a large serving bowl, add everything and gently mix.

Serve immediately.

Nutrition:

Calories 172

Total Fat 11.1 g

Saturated Fat 5.8 g

Cholesterol 610 mg

Sodium 749 mg

Total Carbs 9.9 g

Fiber 2.2 g Sugar 0.2 g

Protein 3.5 g

Cauliflower Hummus

Preparation Time:10 minutes

Cooking Time:0 minutes

Servings: 4

Ingredients:

1 medium head cauliflower, trimmed and chopped

2 garlic cloves, chopped

2 tablespoons of almond butter

2 tablespoons olive oil

1/8 teaspoon ground cumin

Salt, to taste

Pinch of cayenne pepper

Directions:

In a large pan with boiling water, add cauliflower and cook for about 4-5 minutes. Remove from heat and drain well. Keep aside to cool it slightly.

In a food processor, add cauliflower, butter, cumin, and salt and pulse till smooth.

Transfer into a serving bowl. Sprinkle with cayenne pepper and serve immediately.

Nutrition:

Calories 213

Total Fat 8.5 g

Saturated Fat 3.1 g

Cholesterol 120 mg

Sodium 497 mg

Total Carbs 21.4 g

Fiber 0 g

Sugar 0 g Protein 0.1g

CHAPTER 7: DINNER

Tasty Turkey Baked Balls

Preparation Time: 10 minutes

Cooking Time: 30 minutes

Servings: 6

Ingredients:

1 pound ground turkey

½-cup fresh breadcrumbs, white or whole wheat

½-cup Parmesan cheese, freshly grated

½-Tbsp. basil, freshly chopped

½-Tbsp. oregano, freshly chopped

1-pc large egg, beaten

1-Tbsp. parsley, freshly chopped

3-Tbsp.s milk or water

A dash of salt and pepper

A pinch of freshly grated nutmeg

Directions:

Preheat your oven to 350°F.

Line two baking pans with parchment paper.

Stir in all of the ingredients in a large mixing bowl.

Form 1-inch balls from the mixture and place each ball in the baking pan.

Put the pan in the oven.

Bake for 30 minutes, or until the turkey cooks through and the surfaces turn brown.

Turn the meatballs once halfway into the cooking.

Nutrition:

Calories: 517 Cal

Fat: 17.2 g Protein: 38.7 g Carbs: 52.7 g

Fiber: 1 g

Sprouts & Slices In Wheat Wrap

Preparation Time: 10 minutes

Cooking Time: 0 minute

Servings: 2

Ingredients:

¼-cup carrots, grated

½-cup romaine lettuce, shredded

½-pc cucumber, sliced round, then halved

½-cup bean sprouts ¼-cup tomatoes, diced

⅛-cup red onions, diced

¼-cup mozzarella, partly skimmed, shredded

¼-cup hummus or guacamole dressing

1-pc whole-wheat wrap, large

Directions:

In a medium-sized mixing bowl, prepare the dressing or spread by combining all of the ingredients, excluding the cheese and wrap. Mix well until thoroughly combined.

On a clean table, spread out the whole-wheat wrap.

Spread the dressing evenly on the wrap. Be sure to leave a couple of inches on one end of the wrap for folding.

Add the cheese to an even layer over the spread. Fold over the full wrap and tuck in at the bottom.

Nutrition:

Calories: 226 Cal

Fat: 7.5 g

Protein: 16.9 g

Carbs: 27.6 g Fiber: 5 g

Feta-Filled & Tomato-Topped Turkey Burger Bites

Preparation Time: 10 minutes

Cooking Time: 20 minutes

Servings: 1

Ingredients:

1-lb turkey, lean, ground

½-tsp black pepper

Kosher or sea salt to taste

½-cup tomatoes, sun-dried, diced

½-cup Feta cheese, low fat

2-Tbsp.s green onions or chives, diced

Directions:

Stir in all the listed ingredients in a mixing bowl. Mix well until blended thoroughly.

Divide the mixture evenly into four patties. Store them in the refrigerator.

When cooking time comes, you can either grill or fry the frozen patties for about 10 minutes each on both sides.

Serve by topping the burgers with your preferred condiments.

Nutrition:

Calories: 238 Cal

Fat: 7.9 g Protein: 17.8 g

Carbs: 26.8 g

Fiber: 3g

Simply Sautéed Flaky Fillet

Preparation Time: 2 minutes

Cooking Time: 8 minutes

Servings: 6

Ingredients:

6-fillets tilapia

2-Tbsp.s olive oil

1-pc lemon, juice

Salt and pepper to taste

¼-cup parsley or cilantro, chopped

Directions:

Sauté tilapia fillets with olive oil in a medium-sized skillet placed over medium heat. Cook for 4 minutes on each side until the fish flakes easily with a fork.

Add salt and pepper to taste. Pour the lemon juice to each fillet.

To serve, sprinkle the cooked fillets with chopped parsley or cilantro.

Nutrition:

Calories: 249 Cal

Fat: 8.3 g

Protein: 18.6 g

Carbs: 25.9 g

Fiber: 1 g

Spicy Sautéed Chinese Chicken

Preparation Time: 25 minutes

Cooking Time: 5 minutes

Servings: 4

Ingredients:

1-Tbsp. ginger, peeled and minced

1-Tbsp. garlic-chili sauce or chili paste

1-Tbsp. Hoisin sauce 1-Tbsp. light soy sauce

1-lb chicken breasts, boneless, skinless, cubed

1½-Tbsp.s canola oil

Directions:

Whisk all the marinade ingredients altogether in a mixing bowl.

Add in the chicken pieces, and toss lightly to coat the chicken uniformly with the marinade. Cover the bowl.

Chill in the refrigerator for 20 minutes.

Sauté the chicken pieces with canola oil in a medium-sized pan placed over medium-high heat.

Cook for about 5 minutes until its juices run clear and cook through. (Cook further if the chicken pieces are large).

To serve, place the cooked chicken over a choice of either cooked quinoa or brown rice noodles, or brown rice.

Nutrition:

Calories: 190 Cal

Fat: 6.3 g Protein: 14.2 g Carbs: 21 g

Fiber: 2 g

Zesty Zucchini & Chicken In Classic Santa Fe Stir-Fry

Preparation Time: 5 minutes

Cooking Time: 15 minutes

Servings: 2

Ingredients:

1-Tbsp. olive oil

2-pcs chicken breasts, sliced

1-pc onion, small, diced

2-cloves garlic, minced 1-pc zucchini, diced

½- cup carrots, shredded

1-tsp paprika, smoked 1-tsp cumin, ground

½-tsp chili powder ¼-tsp sea salt

2-Tbsp. fresh lime juice

¼-cup cilantro, freshly chopped

Brown rice or quinoa, when serving

Directions:

Sauté the chicken with olive oil for about 3 minutes until the chicken turns brown. Set aside.

Use the same wok and add the onion and garlic.

Cook until the onion is tender.

Add in the carrots and zucchini.

Stir the mixture, and cook further for about a minute.

Add all the seasonings into the mix, and stir to cook for another minute.

Return the chicken in the wok, and pour in the lime juice.

Stir to cook until everything cooks through.

To serve, place the mixture over cooked rice or quinoa and top with the freshly chopped cilantro.

Nutrition:

Calories: 191

Fat: 5.3g

Protein: 11.9g

Carbs: 26.3g

Fiber: 2.5g

Crispy Cheese-Crusted Fish Fillet

Preparation Time: 5 minutes

Cooking Time: 10 minutes

Servings: 4

Ingredients:

¼-cup whole-wheat breadcrumbs

¼-cup Parmesan cheese, grated

¼-tsp sea salt ¼-tsp ground pepper

1-Tbsp. olive oil 4-pcs tilapia fillets

Directions:

Preheat the oven to 375°F.

Stir in the breadcrumbs, Parmesan cheese, salt, pepper, and olive oil in a mixing bowl.

Mix well until blended thoroughly.

Coat the fillets with the mixture, and lay each on a lightly sprayed baking sheet.

Place the sheet in the oven.

Bake for 10 minutes until the fillets cook through and turn brownish.

Nutrition:

Calories: 255

Fat: 7g

Protein: 15.9g

Carbs: 34g

Fiber: 2.6g

Ambrosial Avocado & Salmon Salad in Lemon-Dressed Layers

Preparation Time: 10 minutes

Cooking Time: 0 minute

Servings: 4

Ingredients:

6-oz wild salmon 4-units jars

1-pc avocado, pitted, peeled, and diced

2-cups loosely packed salad greens

½-cup Monterey Jack cheese, reduced-fat, shredded

¾-cup tomato, chopped

1-Tbsp. lemon juice, freshly squeezed

1 Tbsp. lemon juice, freshly squeezed

1 Tbsp. olive oil, extra-virgin

1 tsp honey

⅛-tsp Kosher or sea salt

⅛-tsp black pepper

½-tsp Dijon mustard

Directions:

Combine and whisk all the dressing ingredients, excluding the olive oil in a small mixing bowl.

Mix well.

Drizzle gradually with the oil into the dressing mixture, and keep whisking while pouring.

Pour the dressing as to distribute evenly into each jar.

Distribute uniformly into each jar similar amounts of the following ingredients in this order: diced tomatoes, cheese, avocado, salmon, and lettuce.

Secure each jar by with its lid, and chill the jars in the fridge until ready for serving.

Nutrition:

Calories: 267

Fat: 7.4g

Protein: 16.6g

Carbs: 38.1g

Fiber: 4.8g

Sautéed Shrimp Jambalaya Jumble

Preparation Time: 15 minutes

Cooking Time: 30 minutes

Servings: 4

Ingredients:

10-oz. medium shrimp, peeled

¼-cup celery, chopped ½-cup onion, chopped

1-Tbsp. oil or butter ¼-tsp garlic, minced

¼-tsp onion salt or sea salt

⅓-cup tomato sauce ½-tsp smoked paprika

½-tsp Worcestershire sauce

⅔-cup carrots, chopped

1¼-cups chicken sausage, precooked and diced

2-cups lentils, soaked overnight and precooked

2-cups okra, chopped

A dash of crushed red pepper and black pepper

Parmesan cheese, grated for topping (optional)

Directions:

Sauté the shrimp, celery, and onion with oil in a pan placed over medium-high heat for five minutes, or until the shrimp turn pinkish.

Add in the rest of the ingredients, and sauté further for 10 minutes, or until the veggies are tender.

To serve, divide the jambalaya mixture equally among four serving bowls.

Top with pepper and cheese, if desired.

Nutrition:

Calories: 529

Fat: 17.6g

Protein: 26.4g

Carbs: 98.4g

Fiber: 32.3g

Baked Buffalo Cauliflower Chunks

Preparation Time: 10 minutes

Cooking Time: 35 minutes

Servings: 2

Ingredients:

¼-cup water

¼-cup banana flour

A pinch of salt and pepper

1-pc medium cauliflower, cut into bite-size pieces

½-cup hot sauce

2-Tbsp.s butter, melted

Blue cheese or ranch dressing (optional)

Directions:

Preheat your oven to 425°F. Meanwhile, line a baking pan with foil.

Combine the water, flour, and a pinch of salt and pepper in a large mixing bowl.

Mix well until thoroughly combined.

Add the cauliflower; toss to coat thoroughly.

Transfer the mixture to the baking pan. Bake for 15 minutes, flipping once.

While baking, combine the hot sauce and butter in a small bowl.

Pour the sauce over the baked cauliflower.

Return the baked cauliflower to the oven, and bake further for 20 minutes.

Serve immediately with a ranch dressing on the side, if desired.

Nutrition:

Calories: 168

Cal Fat: 5.6g

Protein: 8.4g

Carbs: 23.8g

Fiber: 2.8g

Cool Garbanzo and Spinach Beans

Preparation Time: 10 minutes

Cooking Time: 0 minute

Servings: 4

Ingredients:

1 tablespoon olive oil

½ onion, diced

10 ounces spinach, chopped

12 ounces garbanzo beans

½ teaspoon cumin

Direction:

Take a skillet and add olive oil, let it warm over medium-low heat

Add onions, garbanzo and cook for 5 minutes

Stir in spinach, cumin, garbanzo beans and season with salt

Use a spoon to smash gently

Cook thoroughly until heated, enjoy!

Nutrition:

Calories: 90

Fat: 4g

Carbohydrates: 11g

Protein: 4g

Lemony Garlic Shrimp

Preparation Time: 10 minutes

Cooking Time: 15 minutes

Servings: 4

Ingredients:

1 and ¼ pounds shrimp, boiled or steamed

3 tablespoons garlic, minced

¼ cup lemon juice

2 tablespoons olive oil

¼ cup parsley

Directions:

Take a small skillet and place it over medium heat, add garlic and oil and stir cook for 1 minute.

Add parsley, lemon juice and season with salt and pepper accordingly.

Add shrimp in a large bowl and transfer the mixture from the skillet over the shrimp.

Chill and serve.

Nutrition:

Calories: 130

Fat: 3g

Carbohydrates: 2g

Protein: 22g

Coconut and Hazelnut Chilled Glass

Preparation Time: 10 minutes

Cooking Time: 0 minute

Servings: 1

Ingredients:

½ cup coconut almond milk

¼ cup hazelnuts, chopped

1 and ½ cups water

1 pack stevia

Directions:

Add listed Ingredients to the blender

Blend until you have a smooth and creamy texture

Serve chilled and enjoy!

Nutrition:

Calories: 457

Fat: 46g

Carbohydrates: 12g

Protein: 7g

Coriander Greens with Zucchini Sauté!

Preparation Time: 10 minutes

Cooking Time: 10 minutes

Servings: 4

Ingredients:

10 ounces beef, sliced into 1-2-inch strips

1 zucchini, cut into 2-inch strips

¼ cup parsley, chopped

3 garlic cloves, minced

2 tablespoons tamari sauce

4 tablespoons avocado oil

Directions:

Add 2 tablespoons avocado oil in a frying pan over high heat

Place strips of beef and brown for a few minutes on high heat

Once the meat is brown, add zucchini strips and Saute until tender

Once tender, add tamari sauce, garlic, parsley and let them sit for a few minutes more
Serve immediately and enjoy!

Nutrition:

Calories: 500

Fat: 40g

Carbohydrates: 5g

Protein: 31g

Walnuts and Asparagus Delight

Preparation Time: 5 minutes

Cooking Time: 5 minutes

Servings: 4

Ingredients:

1 and ½ tablespoons olive oil

¾ pound asparagus, trimmed

¼ cup walnuts, chopped

Sunflower seeds and pepper to taste

Directions:

Place a skillet over medium heat add olive oil and let it heat up.

Add asparagus, Sauté for 5 minutes until browned.

Season with sunflower seeds and pepper.

Remove heat.

Add walnuts and toss.

Nutrition:

Calories: 124

Fat: 12g

Carbohydrates: 2g

Protein: 3g

CHAPTER 8: SALADS AND SOUPS

Green Enchiladas Chicken Soup

Preparation Time: 10 minutes

Cooking Time: 6 hours

Servings: 12

Ingredients:

2½ lbs. chicken thighs or breasts, skinless or boneless

24 oz. chicken broth

28 oz. green enchilada sauce

1 oz. green salsa

1 oz. cubed cream cheese, room temp

Monterey Jack cheese

Pepper and salt to taste

Directions:

Place chicken, chicken broth, and green enchilada sauce into a slow cooker.

Cook for about 6-8 hours on low. Remove the chicken and shred it.

Scoop 1-2 ladles soup into a bowl then stir in half and half. Place back into the slow cooker. Add shredded chicken, green salsa, cream cheese, and jack cheese. Turn your slow cooker to warm, then stir for cheeses to melt. Add more salsa or hot sauce to taste.

Top with topping of choice i.e. cilantro, avocado, sour cream, or green onion.

Nutrition:

Calories: 328

Fats: 19.7g

Carbs: 6g

Protein: 30.8g

Sugars: 2.8g

Fiber: 0.5g

Sodium: 690mg

Potassium: 528mg

Chicken Salsa Soup

Preparation Time: 10 minutes

Cooking Time: 7 hours

Servings: 8

Ingredients:

1 lbs. raw chicken breasts

2 tbsp. Taco seasoning, homemade

Oz cubed cream cheese

1 tbsp. ancho Chile powder

2 tbsp. garlic, minced

1 can green chilies and Rote tomatoes

1 tbsp. salt

½ cup chopped cilantro

½ cup chopped onion

Cups chicken broth

10 oz. riced cauliflower, steamed

1½ cups shredded Mexican blend cheese

Directions:

Layer chicken, taco seasoning, cream cheese, ancho chile powder, garlic, Rotel, salt, cilantro, and onion into a slow cooker.

Pour in chicken broth and cover your slow cooker.

Cook for about 3-4 hours on high or 6-7 hours on low or until chicken falls apart easily and is tender.

Remove the chicken and shred it, then mix well the broth with a whisk. Break apart cream cheese pieces.

Add shredded chicken, cauliflower rice, and shredded cheese. Mix well.

Use toppings of your choice i.e. Avocado, guacamole, extra cheese, or jalapenos. Serve and enjoy.

Nutrition:

Calories: 356

Fat: 17g

Carbs: 6g

Protein: 36g

Sugars: 6g

Fiber: 2g

Sodium: 1680mg

Potassium: 623mg

Beef Vegetable Soup

Preparation Time: 20 minutes

Cooking Time: 3 hours

Servings: 6

Ingredients:

1 tbsp. divided avocado or olive oil

Minced garlic cloves

¾ tbsp. thyme, dried

1½ tbsp. basil, dried

1 tbsp. oregano, dried

½ tbsp. black pepper, ground

¾ tbsp. sea salt

1½ lbs. beef Steak or stew beef, chopped to small pieces

1 small chopped onion

1 chopped red bell pepper

Chopped celery stalks

1x 798ml can tomatoes, diced

½ lb. trimmed green beans, chopped

2 cups beef broth or beef bone stock

Directions:

Heat 1 tbsp. oil in a skillet over medium-high heat.

Meanwhile, combine garlic, thyme, basil, oregano, black pepper, and salt in a bowl, medium, then set aside.

Mix beef and herb blend then sear in the skillet for about 1-2 minutes until golden brown edges.

Transfer the beef into a slow cooker.

Fry onion, pepper, and celery with the remaining oil in the same skillet until onion becomes translucent.

Transfer veggies into your slow cooker then add tomatoes, green beans, and beef stock. Stir to mix.

Cook for about 3-4 hours on high or 5-6 hours on low.

Season with pepper and salt to taste.

Serve and enjoy.

Nutrition:

Calories: 424

Total Fat: 27.7g

Total Carbs: 11.7g

Protein: 33.8g

Sugars: 4.5g

Fiber: 4.7g

Sodium: 1421mg

Potassium: 1315mg

Andouille Sausage Cabbage Soup

Preparation Time: 15 minutes

Cooking Time: 8 hours 15 minutes

Servings: 12

Ingredients:

1 tbsp. virgin olive oil

12 oz andouille sausage, sliced

Cloves garlic, minced

½ cup shallots, chopped

2 cups cabbage, thinly sliced

1 cup cucumbers, chopped

2 cups chicken broth

2 cups water

1 tbsp. apple cider vinegar

1 tbsp. onion powder

Salt to taste

½ tbsp. dried thyme

1 tbsp. caraway seeds

1 tbsp. fennel seeds

Directions:

Grease the skillet with olive oil and heat.

In the skillet, cook sausage together with garlic and shallots until softened and sausage browned.

Add the sausage mixture in a slow cooker alongside the remaining ingredients.

Cook covered on low for 8 hours.

Serve warm and enjoy

Nutrition:

Calories 132

Total Fat: 9g

Total Carbs: 4g

Protein: 6g

Sugar: 2g

Fiber: 1g

Sodium: 898mg

Potassium: 294mg

Broccoli Cheese Soup

Preparation Time: 10 minutes

Cooking Time: 3 hours 10 minutes

Servings: 12

Ingredients:

1 tbsp. softened butter, unsalted

5 oz cream cheese, softened

1 cup whipping cream

2 cups of chicken broth (warmed in microwave)

2 cups water

½ cup Parmesan cheese

2 cups fresh broccoli, chopped

Dash of thyme

2 ½ cups cheddar cheese, shredded

Salt and pepper to taste

Directions:

In the slow cooker, add butter, cream cheese, whipping cream, chicken broth, water and stir well.

When perfectly mixed pour in the Parmesan cheese.

In the cooker, add chopped broccoli and thyme.

Cover the cooker and cook on low for 3 hours.

Perfectly mix the soup, then add cheddar cheese and mix for a while for the cheddar cheese to melt fully.

Add salt and pepper to taste.

When fully mixed, thin out the soup by adding some water or chicken broth.

Serve and enjoy!

Nutrition:

Calories 230

Total Fat: 20g

Total Carbs: 3.8g

Protein: 9.8

Sugar: 0.9g

Fiber: 1g

Sodium: 370mg

Loaded Cauliflower Soup

Preparation Time: 10 minutes

Cooking Time: 8 hours

Servings: 6

Ingredients:

1 cup celery, chopped

2 cups cauliflower, cut into florets

1 cup cucumber

3 cups chicken stocks

1 tbsp. garlic powder,

1 tbsp. bullion

1 tbsp. salt

1 tbsp. onion powder

1 tbsp. parsley flakes

½ cup heavy cream

1 ½ tbsp. butter

1 lb. bottom round steak

Directions:

Slice the celery into pieces then add them together with cauliflowers, cucumbers, and chicken in your slow cooker.

Add 3 tbsp. garlic, bullion, and 2 tbsp. seasoning salt, onion powder, and parsley flakes, then turn on high for 4-5 hours or low for 8-10 hours.

When halfway through with cooking, vegetables will be tender, so add heavy cream. Using an immersion blender, puree your soup.

In a pan heat butter over medium-high heat, slice the steak into ½ inch cubes then season with garlic powder and salt.

Fry your steak in the pan with butter and add them in your slow cooker then continue cooking until ready.

Serve with bacon, sour cream, and shredded cheese as desired and enjoy.

Nutrition:

Calories 400

Fat 26g

Carbs 17g

Protein 23g

Sugar 7g

Fiber 3g

Sodium 410mg

Potassium 790mg

Chicken Tortilla Soup

Preparation Time: 10 minutes

Cooking Time: 4 hours

Servings: 4

Ingredients:

2 lbs. chicken thighs, boneless and skinless,

1 cup salsa, low-carb

1 cup heavy whipping cream

1 tbsp. salt

2 tbsp. adobo seasoning

5oz shredded Colby-jack cheese

5oz shredded pepper jack cheese

2 cups chicken broth

1 tbsp. xanthan gum

Whole-wheat tortillas

2 tbsp. butter

Directions:

Place chicken thighs, salsa, cream, salt, and adobo seasoning in the slow cooker.

Cook for 4 hours on low or until chicken is cooked completely.

Shred your chicken and add it back to your slow cooker.

Add half of the cheeses and pour in chicken broth.

To get a thicker soup, add in 1 tbsp. of xanthan gum, and cook on low until cheeses melt; about one hour more.

Make tortilla strips while the soup is cooking by slicing shells into strips.

Dredge butter through and place on a pan, then bake for 10-15 minutes on 350 degrees, be careful not to burn.

Serve your soup with tortilla strips and remaining cheeses.

Nutrition:

Calories 619g

Fat 48g

Carbs 7g

Protein 40g

Sugar 4g

Fiber 1g

Sodium 256mg

Potassium 118mg

Cooker Broccoli Soup

Preparation Time: 15minutes

Cooking Time: 2 hours 30 minutes

Servings: 4

Ingredients:

2 cups broccoli

½ cup heavy whipping cream

2 cups chicken broth

¼ cup cream cheese, cut into ½ inch squares,

¼ cup butter

1 ¾ cop cheddar cheese

¾ cup mozzarella cheese

Pepper and salt (to taste)

Directions:

Place broccoli into your slow cooker, then, add whipping cream and chicken broth.

Add cream cheese and butter in the slow cooker.

Cover the slow cooker and cook for 1 ½ hour on high.

Stir your mixture and cover it with cheddar cheese and mozzarella, continue stirring until cheese incorporates.

Cook for 1 hour, then add pepper and salt to taste.

Nutrition:

Calories 647

Fat 54.6g

Carbs 10.2g

Protein 31.5g

Fiber 3g

Sodium 1151mg

Potassium 585mg

Chicken Chili Soup

Preparation Time: 5 minutes

Cooking Time: 6 hours

Servings: 8

Ingredients:

2 tbsp. butter, unsalted,

1 pepper

1 onion

1 tbsp. thyme

5 chicken thighs

8 pieces of bacon, sliced,

1 tbsp. coconut flour

1 tbsp. garlic, minced,

1 tbsp. salt

1 tbsp. pepper

1 cup chicken stock

2 tbsp. lemon juice

¼ cup coconut milk, unsweetened

2 tbsp. tomato paste

Directions:

Place butter pats at the center of your slow cooker.

Thinly dice peppers and onions then disperse them evenly on the bottom of your slow cooker.

Cover with chicken thighs.

Distribute your bacon slices over the chicken.

Add coconut flour, garlic, salt, and pepper.

Pour in chicken stock, lemon juice, coconut milk, and tomato paste.

Cook for 6 hours on low.

Breakup chicken, stir, then serve and enjoy.

Nutrition:

Calories 470

Fat 38g

Carbs 6g

Protein 27g

Sugar 2g

Fiber 1g

Sodium 720mg

Potassium 460mg

Stuffed Pepper Soup

Preparation Time: 15 minutes

Cooking Time: 8 hours 5minutes Serves 8

Ingredients:

1 lb. ground beef

2 tbsp. onion, dried and minced

1 tbsp. garlic, minced

Salt and pepper to taste

3 cups beef broth

24 oz. marinara sauce

1 cup rice cauliflower

2 cups chopped bell pepper

½ tbsp. oregano

½ tbsp. basil

Shredded mozzarella

Directions:

Sauté the beef, garlic, and onion in a skillet until browned then transfer to a slow cooker.

Stir in salt and pepper, beef broth, marinara sauce, riced cauliflower, bell pepper, oregano, and basil to the slow cooker.

Cover the slow cooker and cook for 8 hours.

Garnish with shredded mozzarella.

Serve and enjoy.

Nutrition:

Calories 193

Fat 12g

Carbs 9g

Protein 13g

Sugar: 6g

Fiber: 3g

Sodium: 826mg

Potassium 642g

Chicken Avocado Soup

Preparation Time: 10 minutes

Cooking Time: 4 hours

Servings: 4

Ingredients:

1 lb. chicken breast, skinless

2 cups chicken broth, low sodium

2 cups of water

5 sliced scallions

1 diced Roma tomato

1 sliced celery stalks

2 minced garlic cloves

1 tbsp. salt

1 tbsp. coriander

½ tbsp. cumin

¼ tbsp. pepper

1 tbsp. lime juice

2 sliced avocados, pitted and peeled

2 tbsp. cilantro, fresh

Directions:

Add chicken breast, chicken broth, water, scallions, Roma tomato, celery stalks, garlic cloves, Salt, coriander, Cumin, pepper, and lime juice to a slow cooker.

Stir the ingredients until well combined.

Cover the slow cooker and cook for 4 hours.

Transfer the chicken to a chopping board and shred it using two forks.

Add back the chicken to the slow cooker and cook for another fifteen minutes.

Use a ladle to serve the soup into bowls.

Add a few slices of avocado to the soup and garnish it with cilantro.

Enjoy your soup.

Nutrition:

Calories 196,

Total Fat 9.7g

Carbs 7.9g

Protein 20.3g

Sugar: 2.6g

Fiber: 3.8g

CHAPTER 9: DESSERTS

Blueberry-Peach Cobbler

Preparation Time: 15 minutes

Cooking Time: 2 hours

Servings: 4

Ingredients:

5 tablespoons coconut oil, divided

3 large peaches, peeled and sliced

2 cups frozen blueberries

1 cup almond flour

1 cup rolled oats

1 tablespoon maple syrup

1 tablespoon coconut sugar

1 teaspoon ground cinnamon

½ teaspoon vanilla extract

Pinch ground nutmeg

Directions:

Coat the bottom of your slow cooker with 1 tablespoon of coconut oil.

Arrange the peaches and blueberries along the bottom of the slow cooker.

In a small bowl, stir together the almond flour, oats, remaining 4 tablespoons of coconut oil, maple syrup, coconut sugar, cinnamon, vanilla, and nutmeg until a coarse mixture forms.

Gently crumble the topping over the fruit in the slow cooker.

Cover the cooker and set to high. Cook for 2 hours and serve.

Nutrition:

Calories: 516

Total Fat: 34g

Total Carbs: 49g

Sugar: 24g

Fiber: 10g

Protein: 10g

Sodium: 1mg

Chai Spice Baked Apples

Preparation Time: 15 minutes

Cooking Time: 3 hours

Servings: 5

Ingredients:

5 apples

½ cup water

½ cup crushed pecans (optional)

¼ cup melted coconut oil

1 teaspoon ground cinnamon

½ teaspoon ground ginger

¼ teaspoon ground cardamom

¼ teaspoon ground cloves

Directions:

Core each apple, and peel off a thin strip from the top of each.

Add the water to the slow cooker. Gently place each apple upright along the bottom.

In a small bowl, stir together the pecans (if using), coconut oil, cinnamon, ginger, cardamom, and cloves.

Drizzle the mixture over the tops of the apples.

Cover the cooker and set to high. Cook for 2 to 3 hours, until the apples soften, and serve.

Nutrition:

Calories: 217

Total Fat: 12g

Total Carbs: 30g

Sugar: 22g Fiber: 6g Protein: 0g
Sodium: 0mg

Protein: 18g
Sodium: 665mg

Cacao Brownies

Preparation Time: 15 minutes

Cooking Time: 3 hours

Servings: 4

Ingredients:

3 tablespoons coconut oil, divided

1 cup almond butter

1 cup unsweetened cacao powder

½ cup coconut sugar

2 large eggs

2 ripe bananas

2 teaspoons vanilla extract

1 teaspoon baking soda

½ teaspoon sea salt

Directions:

Coat the bottom of the slow cooker with 1 tablespoon of coconut oil.

In a medium bowl, combine the almond butter, cacao powder, coconut sugar, eggs, bananas, vanilla, baking soda, and salt

Mash the bananas and stir well until a batter forms

Pour the batter into the slow cooker.

Cover the cooker and set to low. Cook for 2½ to 3 hours, until firm to a light touch but still gooey in the middle, and serve.

Nutrition:

Calories: 779

Total Fat: 51g

Total Carbs: 68g

Sugar: 35g

Fiber: 15g

Cinnamon Pecans

Preparation Time: 15 minutes

Cooking Time: 4 hours

Servings: 3 ½ cups

Ingredients:

1 tablespoon coconut oil

1 large egg white

2 tablespoons ground cinnamon

2 teaspoons vanilla extract

¼ cup maple syrup

2 tablespoons coconut sugar

¼ teaspoon sea salt

3 cups pecan halves

Directions:

Coat the slow cooker with the coconut oil.

In a medium bowl, whisk the egg white.

Add the cinnamon, vanilla, maple syrup, coconut sugar, and salt. Whisk well to combine.

Add the pecans and stir to coat. Pour the pecans into the slow cooker.

Cover the cooker and set to low. Cook for 3 to 4 hours.

Remove the pecans from the slow cooker and spread them on a baking sheet or another cooling surface.

Let cool for 5 to 10 minutes before serving.

Store in an airtight container at room temperature for up to 2 weeks.

Nutrition:

Calories: 195

Total Fat: 18g

Total Carbs: 9g

Sugar: 6g

Fiber: 3g

Protein: 2g

Sodium: 46mg

Missouri Haystack Cookies

Preparation Time: 15 minutes

Cooking Time: 1 ½ hours

Servings: 24 pieces

Ingredients:

½ cup coconut oil

½ cup unsweetened almond milk

1 overripe banana, mashed well

½ cup coconut sugar

¼ cup cacao powder

1 teaspoon vanilla extract

¼ teaspoon sea salt

3 cups rolled oats

½ cup almond butter

Directions:

In a medium bowl, stir together the coconut oil, almond milk, mashed banana, coconut sugar, cacao powder, vanilla, and salt.

Pour the mixture into the slow cooker.

Pour the oats on top without stirring.

Put the almond butter on top of the oats without stirring.

Cover the cooker and set to high. Cook for 1½ hours.

Stir the mixture well. As it cools, scoop tablespoon-size balls out and press onto a baking sheet to continue to cool. Serve when hardened.

Keep leftovers refrigerated in an airtight container for up to 1 week.

Nutrition:

Calories: 140

Total Fat: 9g

Total Carbs: 14g

Sugar: 5g

Fiber: 2g

Protein: 2g

Sodium: 29mg

Coconut-Vanilla Yogurt

Preparation Time: 15 minutes

Cooking Time: 2 hours, overnight to ferment

Servings: 3 ½ cups

Ingredients:

3 (13.5-ounce) cans full-fat coconut milk

5 probiotic capsules (not pills)

1 teaspoon raw honey

½ teaspoon vanilla extract

Directions:

Pour the coconut milk into the slow cooker. Cover the cooker and set to high. Cook for 1 to 2 hours, until the temperature of the milk reaches 180ºF measured with a candy thermometer.

Turn off the slow cooker and allow the temperature of the milk to come down close to 100ºF.

Open the probiotic capsules and pour in the contents, along with the honey and vanilla. Stir well to combine.

Re-cover the slow cooker, turn it off and unplug it, and wrap it in an insulating towel to keep warm overnight as it ferments. Pour the yogurt into sterilized jars and refrigerate. The yogurt should thicken slightly in the refrigerator, where it will keep for up to 1 week.

Nutrition:

Calories: 305
Total Fat: 30g
Total Carbs: 7g
Sugar: 3g
Fiber: 0g
Protein: 2g
Sodium: 43mg

Salted Dark Drinking Chocolate

Preparation Time: 15 minutes

Cooking Time: 4 hours

Servings: 4 cups

Ingredients:

5 cups unsweetened almond milk
2½ tablespoons coconut oil
5 tablespoons cacao powder
5 cinnamon sticks
3 to 4 teaspoons coconut sugar or raw honey
1 tablespoon vanilla extract
1 (3-inch) piece fresh ginger
1 (2-inch) piece turmeric root
3 tablespoons collagen peptides
½ to ¾ teaspoon sea salt, divided

Directions:

In your slow cooker, combine the almond milk, coconut oil, cacao powder, cinnamon sticks, coconut sugar or honey, vanilla, ginger, and turmeric.

Cover the cooker and set to low. Cook for 3 to 4 hours.

Pour the contents of the cooker through a fine-mesh sieve into a clean container; discard the solids.

Stir in the collagen peptides until well combined.

Pour the chocolate into mugs and gently sprinkle ⅛ teaspoon of sea salt on top of each beverage. Serve hot.

Nutrition:

Calories: 235
Total Fat: 14g
Total Carbs: 20g
Sugar: 12g
Fiber: 4g
Protein: 7g
Sodium: 512mg

Warm Cinnamon-Turmeric Almond Milk

Preparation Time: 15 minutes

Cooking Time: 4 hours

Servings: 4

Ingredients:

4 cups unsweetened almond milk
4 cinnamon sticks
2 tablespoons coconut oil
1 (4-inch) piece turmeric root, roughly chopped
1 (2-inch) piece fresh ginger, roughly chopped
1 teaspoon raw honey, plus more to taste

Directions:

In your slow cooker, combine the almond milk, cinnamon sticks, coconut oil, turmeric, and ginger.

Cover the cooker and set to low. Cook for 3 to 4 hours.

Pour the contents of the cooker through a fine-mesh sieve into a clean container; discard the solids.

Starting with just 1 teaspoon, add raw honey to taste.

Nutrition:

Calories: 133
Total Fat: 11g
Total Carbs: 10g
Sugar: 7g
Fiber: 1g Protein: 1g Sodium: 152mg

Café-Style Fudge

Preparation Time: 10 minutes

Cooking Time: 0 minute

Servings: 6

Ingredients:

1 tablespoon instant coffee granules
4 tablespoons confectioners' Swerve
4 tablespoons cocoa powder
1 stick butter
1/2 teaspoon vanilla extract

Directions:

Beat the butter and Swerve at low speed. Add in the cocoa powder, instant coffee granules, and vanilla and continue to mix until well combined.

Spoon the batter into a foil-lined baking sheet. Refrigerate for 2 to 3 hours. Enjoy!

Nutrition:

Calories: 144
Fat: 15.5g
Carbs: 2.1g
Protein: .8g
Fiber: 1.1g

Coconut and Seed Porridge

Preparation Time: 15 minutes

Cooking Time: 20 minutes

Servings: 2

Ingredients:

6 tablespoons coconut flour

1/2 cup canned coconut milk

4 tablespoons double cream

2 tablespoons flaxseed meal

1 tablespoon pumpkin seeds, ground

Directions:

In a saucepan, simmer all of the above the ingredients over medium-low heat. Add in a keto sweetener of choice.

Divide the porridge between bowls and enjoy!

Nutrition:

Calories: 300

Fat: 25.1g

Carbs: 8g

Protein: 4.9

Fiber: 6g

Pecan and Lime Cheesecake

Preparation Time: 30 minutes

Cooking Time: 0 minute

Servings: 10

Ingredients:

1 cup coconut flakes

20 ounces mascarpone cheese, room temperature

1 ½ cups pecan meal

1/2 cup xylitol

3 tablespoons key lime juice

Directions:

Combine the pecan meal, 1/4 cup of xylitol, and coconut flakes in a mixing bowl. Press the crust into a parchment-lined springform pan. Freeze for 30 minutes.

Now, beat the mascarpone cheese with 1/4 cup of xylitol with an electric mixer.

Beat in the key lime juice; you can add vanilla extract if desired.

Spoon the filling onto the prepared crust. Allow it to cool in your refrigerator for about 3 hours. Bon appétit!

Nutrition:

Calories: 296

Fat: 20g

Carbs: 6g

Protein: 21g

Fiber: 3.7g

Rum Butter Cookies

Preparation Time: 10 minutes

Cooking Time: 0 minute

Servings: 12

Ingredients:

1/2 cup coconut butter

1 teaspoon rum extract

4 cups almond meal

1 stick butter

1/2 cup confectioners' Swerve

Directions:

Melt the coconut butter and butter. Stir in the Swerve and rum extract.

Afterward, add in the almond meal and mix to combine.

Roll the balls and place them on a parchment-lined cookie sheet. Place in your refrigerator until ready to serve.

Nutrition:

Calories: 400

Fats: 40g

Carbs: 4.9g

Protein: 5.4g

Fiber: 2.9g

Fluffy Chocolate Chip Cookies

Preparation Time: 10 minutes

Cooking Time: 0 minute

Servings: 10

Ingredients:

1/2 cup almond meal

4 tablespoons double cream

1/2 cup sugar-free chocolate chips

2 cups coconut, unsweetened and shredded

1/2 cup monk fruit syrup

Directions:

In a mixing bowl, combine all of the above ingredients until well combined. Shape the batter into bite-sized balls.

Flatten the balls using a fork or your hand.

Place in your refrigerator until ready to serve.

Nutrition:

Calories: 109

Fats: 9.5g

Carbs: 4.1g

Protein: 2.1g

Fiber: 2.6g

Chewy Almond Blondies

Preparation Time: 55 minutes

Cooking Time: 0 minute

Servings: 10

Ingredients:

1/2 cup sugar-free bakers' chocolate, chopped into small chunks

1/4 cup erythritol

2 tablespoons coconut oil

1 cup almond meal

1 cup almond butter

Directions:

In a mixing bowl, combine almond meal, almond butter, and erythritol until creamy and uniform.

Press the mixture into a foil-lined baking sheet. Freeze for 30 to 35 minutes.

Melt the coconut oil and bakers' chocolate to make the glaze. Spread the glaze over your cake; freeze until the chocolate is set.

Slice into bars and devour!

Nutrition:

Calories: 234

Fats: 25.1g

Carbs: 3.6g

Protein: 1.7g

Fiber: 1.4g

Fluffy Chocolate Crepes

Preparation Time: 20 minutes

Cooking Time: 20 minutes

Servings: 2

Ingredients:

1/4 cup coconut milk, unsweetened

2 egg, beaten

1/2 cup coconut flour

1 tablespoon unsweetened cocoa powder

2 tablespoons coconut oil, melted

Directions:

In a mixing bowl, thoroughly combine the coconut flour and cocoa powder along with 1/2 teaspoon of baking soda.

In another bowl, whisk the eggs and coconut milk. Add the flour mixture to the egg mixture; mix to combine well.

In a frying pan, preheat 1 tablespoon of the coconut oil until sizzling. Ladle 1/2 of the batter into the frying pan and cook for 2 to 3 minutes on each side.

Melt the remaining tablespoon of coconut oil and fry another crepe for about 5 minutes. Serve with your favorite keto filling. Bon appétit!

Nutrition:

Calories: 330
Fats: 31.9g
Carbs: 7.1g
Protein: 7.3g - Fiber: 3.5g

CHAPTER 10: SIDES

Chili Cauliflower Rice

Preparation Time: 10 minutes

Cooking Time: 20 minutes

Servings: 6

Ingredients:

1 cup chopped yellow onion

3 tablespoons olive oil

2 cups riced cauliflower

¾ cup crushed tomatoes

2 garlic cloves, minced

2 cups veggie stock

¼ cup chopped cilantro

½ teaspoon chili powder

Directions:

Heat up a pan with the oil over medium-high heat and add the onions and garlic. Stir and cook for 4 minutes.

Add cauliflower rice, stock, salt, pepper tomatoes and chili powder then stir, cook for 15 minutes and take off the heat.

Add the cilantro and mix briefly, then divide between plates and serve.

Enjoy!

Nutrition:

Calories: 200

Fat: 4g

Fiber: 3g

Carbs: 6g

Protein: 8g

90. Herbed Quinoa

Preparation Time: 10 minutes

Cooking Time: 15 minutes

Servings: 4

Ingredients:

2 cups quinoa

3 cups water

Juice of 1 lemon

A pinch of salt and black pepper

A handful mixed parsley, cilantro and basil, chopped

Directions:

In a pot, mix the quinoa with water, lemon, salt and pepper.

Bring to a boil and simmer over medium heat for 15 minutes.

Take off the heat, add mixed herbs, stir and set aside for 10 minutes.

Once cooled slightly, fluff with a fork, divide between plates and serve as a side dish.

Nutrition:

Calories: 202

Fat: 1g

Fiber: 6g

Carbs: 12g

Protein: 10g

Black Beans and Veggie Mix

Preparation Time: 10 minutes

Cooking Time: 1 hour and 5 minutes

Servings: 6

Ingredients:

1 teaspoon olive oil

16 ounces black beans, soaked and drained

12 ounces green bell pepper, chopped

12 ounces sweet onion, chopped

4 garlic cloves, minced

2 ½ teaspoons ground cumin

2 tablespoons tomato paste

2 quarts water

A pinch of salt and black pepper

Directions:

Heat up a pot with the oil over medium-high heat and add the onion, bell pepper and garlic. Stir and cook for 5 minutes.

Add the beans, cumin, tomato paste, salt, pepper and the water.

Toss, bring to a simmer, reduce heat to medium and cook the beans mix for 1 hour. Divide between plates and serve as a side dish.

Nutrition:

Calories 221

Fat 5g - Fiber 4g

Carbs 9g - Protein 11g

Green Beans and Mushroom Sauté

Preparation Time: 10 minutes

Cooking Time: 25 minutes

Servings: 6

Ingredients:

1 pound green beans, trimmed

8 ounces white mushrooms, sliced

1 yellow onion, chopped

2 tablespoons olive oil

½ cup veggie stock

A pinch of salt and black pepper

Directions:

Heat up a big pan with the oil over medium-high heat and add the onion, stir and cook for 4 minutes.

Add the stock and the mushrooms, then stir and cook for 6 minutes more.

Add green beans, salt and pepper.

Toss and cook over medium heat for 15 minutes, then divide everything between plates and serve as a side dish.

Nutrition:

Calories 182

Fat 4g

Fiber 5g

Carbs 6g

Protein 8g

Cauliflower Mash

Preparation Time: 10 minutes

Cooking Time: 15 minutes

Servings: 4

Ingredients:

1½ cups veggie stock

1 cauliflower head, florets separated

2 teaspoons olive oil

A pinch of salt and black pepper

½ teaspoon ground turmeric

3 chives, chopped

Directions:

Put the stock and the cauliflower in a pot and bring to a boil over medium heat.

Cook for 15 minutes, drain, and transfer to a bowl then mash using a potato masher.

Add the oil, salt, pepper, chives and turmeric.

Stir really well, divide between plates and serve as a side dish.

Nutrition:

Calories 200

Fat 4g

Fiber 6g

Carbs 7g

Protein 10g

Creamy Rice

Preparation Time: 10 minutes

Cooking Time: 20 minutes

Servings: 4

Ingredients:

14 ounces coconut milk

1½ cups jasmine rice

1 tablespoon coconut cream

½ cup water

A pinch of salt and white pepper

Directions:

In a pot, mix the rice with the coconut milk, coconut cream, water, salt and white pepper. Stir and bring to a simmer over medium heat for 20 minutes.

Stir one more time then divide between plates and serve as a side dish.

Nutrition:

Calories 191

Fat 5g

Fiber 4g

Carbs 11g

Protein 9g

Mushroom and Cauliflower Rice

Preparation Time: 10 minutes

Cooking Time: 15 minutes

Servings: 6

Ingredients:

1½ cups cauliflower rice

2 tablespoons olive oil

4 ounces wild mushrooms, roughly chopped

3 shallots, chopped

8 ounces cremini mushrooms, roughly chopped

2 cups veggie stock

A pinch of salt and black pepper

2 tablespoons chopped cilantro

Directions:

Heat up a pot with the oil over medium heat and add the cauliflower rice and shallots. Stir and cook for 5 minutes.

Add stock, cremini mushrooms and wild mushrooms, then stir and cook for 10 minutes more.

Add the parsley, salt and pepper and mix. Divide between plates and serve.

Nutrition:

Calories 189

Fat 3g - Fiber 4g

Carbs 9g - Protein 8g

Simple Broccoli Stir-Fry

Preparation Time: 10 minutes

Cooking Time: 12 minutes

Servings: 4

Ingredients:

6 garlic cloves, minced

1 broccoli head, florets separated

½ cup veggie stock

1 tablespoon olive oil

1 tablespoon balsamic vinegar

A pinch of salt and black pepper

Directions:

Heat up a pan with the oil over medium heat, add the garlic, stir and cook for 5 minutes.

Add the broccoli, stock, vinegar, salt and pepper.

Mix and cook for 7-8 minutes more, then divide between plates and serve as a side dish.

Nutrition:

Calories 182

Fat 6g

Fiber 3g

Carbs 8g

Protein 6g

Glazed Baby Carrots

Preparation Time: 10 minutes

Cooking Time: 15 minutes

Servings: 4

Ingredients:

1 tablespoon olive oil

3 pounds baby carrots, peeled

1 tablespoon maple syrup

1 teaspoon thyme, dried

1 tablespoon mustard

2 tablespoons veggie stock

Directions:

Heat up a pan with the oil over medium heat, add the baby carrots and brown them for 5-6 minutes.

Add the maple syrup, thyme, stock and mustard, mix and cook for 10 minutes more. Divide between plates and serve.

Nutrition:

Calories 180,

Fat 6g

Fiber 7g

Carbs 15g

Protein 6g

Baked Asparagus

Preparation Time: 10 minutes

Cooking Time: 15 minutes

Servings: 4

Ingredients:

5 tablespoons olive oil

4 garlic cloves, minced

2 tablespoons chopped shallot

Black pepper to the taste

1½ teaspoons balsamic vinegar

1½ pound asparagus, trimmed

Directions:

Spread the asparagus on a lined baking sheet, and drizzle the oil.

Add the garlic, shallot, vinegar and black pepper, then toss well and place in the oven.

Bake at 450 degrees F for 15 minutes.

Divide between plates and serve as a side dish.

Nutrition:

Calories 132

Fat 1g

Fiber 2g

Carbs 4g

Protein 4g

Cucumber Salad

Preparation Time: 1 hour

Cooking Time: 0 minutes

Servings: 12

Ingredients:

2 cucumbers, chopped

2 tomatoes, chopped

1 tablespoon olive oil

1 yellow onion, chopped

1 jalapeno pepper, chopped

1 garlic clove, minced

1 teaspoon chopped parsley

2 tablespoons lime juice

2 teaspoons chopped cilantro

½ teaspoon dill, dried

Directions:

In a large salad bowl, mix the cucumbers with the tomatoes, onion, jalapeno, garlic, parsley, lime juice, cilantro, dill and oil.

Mix well and keep in the fridge for 1 hour before serving as a side salad.

Nutrition:

Calories 132

Fat 3g

Fiber 1g

Carbs 7g

Protein 4g

Eggplant Side Salad

Preparation Time: 10 minutes

Cooking Time: 10 minutes

Servings: 6

Ingredients:

1/3 cup homemade mayonnaise

2 tablespoons balsamic vinegar

A pinch of salt and black pepper

1 tablespoon lime juice

2 big eggplants, sliced

¼ cup chopped parsley

¼ cup avocado oil

Directions:

In a small bowl, mix mayonnaise with vinegar, lime juice and black pepper. Stir well and set aside.

Brush each eggplant slice with the avocado oil and season with salt and pepper.

Place on the preheated grill over medium-high heat, and cook for 5 minutes on each side.

Divide between plates.

Drizzle the mayo mix all over, sprinkle parsley and serve as a side dish.

Nutrition:

Calories 180

Fat 2g

Fiber 2g

Carbs 8g

Protein 6g

Barley Mix

Preparation Time: 10 minutes

Cooking Time: 45 minutes

Servings: 4

Ingredients:

1 tablespoon olive oil

1 yellow onion, chopped

4 parsnips, roughly chopped

1 tablespoon chopped sage

1 garlic clove, minced

14 ounces barley

6 cups hot veggie stock

Salt and black pepper

Directions:

Heat up a pan with the oil over medium-high heat and add onion. Stir and cook for 5 minutes.

Add parsnips, sage, garlic, barley and stock. Stir well, bring to a simmer and cook for 40 minutes.

Divide between plates and serve.

Nutrition:

Calories 286

Fat 4g

Fiber 9g

Carbs 29g

Protein 4g

Lentil and Chickpea Salad

Preparation Time: 15 minutes

Cooking Time: 30 minutes

Servings: 4

Ingredients:

7 ounces lentils, rinsed

3 tablespoons chopped capers

Juice of 1 lemon

Zest of 1 lemon

1 red onion, chopped

3 tablespoons olive oil

16 ounces canned chickpeas, drained

1 tablespoon chopped parsley

A pinch of salt and black pepper

Directions:

Put lentils in a pot, add water to cover and bring to a simmer over medium heat.

Boil for 30 minutes, drain and transfer to a bowl.

Add capers, lemon juice, lemon zest, onion, oil, chickpeas, parsley, salt and pepper, toss and serve as a side dish.

Nutrition:

Calories 212

Fat 4g

Fiber 4g

Carbs 12g

Protein 6g

Rice and Beans

Preparation Time: 10 minutes

Cooking Time: 1 hour

Servings: 6

Ingredients:

1 tablespoon olive oil

1 yellow onion, chopped

2 celery stalks, chopped

2 garlic cloves, minced

2 cups brown rice

1½ cup canned black beans, rinsed and drained

4 cups veggie stock

Salt and black pepper to the taste

Directions:

Heat up a pan with the olive oil over medium heat, add celery and onion.

Stir and cook for 8 minutes.

Add beans and garlic, stir again and sauté them as well for about 5 minutes.

Add rice, stock, salt and pepper. Stir, cover, cook for 45 minutes, then divide between plates and serve.

Nutrition:

Calories 212

Fat 3g

Fiber 2g

Carbs 2g

Protein 1g

CHAPTER 11: DRINKS AND SMOOTHIES

Berry Smoothie

Preparation Time: 5 minutes

Cooking Time: 0 minute

Servings: 2

Ingredients:

300ml Cups Apple

1 Banana

350g Frozen Berries

170g Sour Yoghurt

1 Tbsp. Honey

Berries

Directions:

Mix everything in a blender except the berries until smooth.

Garnish with fresh berries.

Nutrition:

Calories: 221kcal

Carbohydrates: 52g

Protein: 6g

Fat: 1g

Pineapple Turmeric Smoothie

Preparation Time: 5 minutes

Cooking Time: 0 minute

Servings: 2

Ingredients:

1 Banana

400g Frozen Pineapple

1/4 Cup Coconut Milk

1/4 Tbsp. Turmeric Powder

Directions:

Blend everything.

Garnish with lemon zest.

Nutrition:

Calories: 327 kcal

Carbs: 48 g

Fat: 14 g

Protein: 2 g

Wild Berry Smoothie

Preparation Time: 5 minutes

Cooking Time: 0 minute

Servings: 2

Ingredients:

350g Frozen Wild Berries

200g Sour Yoghurt

1 tbsp. Brown Sugar

4/5 Ice Cubes

Directions:

Blend everything.

Serve with berries.

Nutrition:

Calories: 334 kcal

Carbs: 34 g

Fat: 4.3 g

Protein: 1.2 g

Strawberry Smoothie

Preparation Time: 5 minutes

Cooking Time: 0 minute

Servings: 2

Ingredients:

300ml Sour Yoghurt

200g Frozen Strawberries

1 Banana

2 Tbsp. Brown Sugar

3 Strawberries

Directions:

Blend everything.

Serve with strawberries.

Nutrition:

Calories:371 kcal

Carbs: 51 g

Fat: 4.2 g

Protein: 1.4 g

Avocado Smoothie

Preparation Time: 5 minutes

Cooking Time: 0 minute

Servings: 2

Ingredients:

1 Large Avocado (Peeled)

1 Cup Golden Milk

1/8 Tbsp. Vanilla Extract

2 Tbsp. Maple Syrup

Salt

Directions:

Blend everything.

Add ice cubes.

Nutrition:

Calories: 323.2 kcal

Carbs: 29.2 g

Fat: 25.1 g

Protein: 5.1 g

Apple Smoothie

Preparation Time: 5 minutes

Cooking Time: 0 minute

Servings: 2

Ingredients:

2 Cup Apple(Chopped)

200ml Sour Yoghurt

1/2 Cup Frozen Banana(Chopped)

1 Tbsp. Maple Syrup

1/8 Tbsp. Cinnamon Powder

3/4 Ice Cubes

Mint Leaves

Directions:

Blend everything.

Add ice cubes.

Nutrition:

Calories: 305 kcal

Carbs: 53 g

Fat: 2 g

Protein: 6 g

Papaya Smoothie

Preparation Time: 5 minutes

Cooking Time: 0 minute

Servings: 2

Ingredients:

250ml Golden Milk

200gm Ripe Papaya Puree

1/8 Tbsp. Cinnamon Powder

1 Cup Frozen Banana (Chopped)

1 Cup Plain Yoghurt

1 Tbsp. Lemon Juice

Directions:

Blend everything and serve.

Nutrition:

Calories: 224.5 kcal

Carbs: 33.7 g

Fat: 7.7g

Protein: 6.9 g

Kiwi Smoothie

Preparation Time: 5 minutes

Cooking Time: 0 minute

Servings: 2

Ingredients:

300g Peeled Frozen Kiwi Fruit

1 Cup Frozen Chopped Mango

300ml Apple Juice

1 Banana

1 Kiwi

Directions:

Blend everything.

Garnish with kiwi

Nutrition:

Calories: 285 kcal

Carbs: 51 g

Fat: 9 g

Protein: 6 g

Coconut Turmeric Smoothie

Preparation Time: 5 minutes

Cooking Time: 0 minute

Servings: 2

Ingredients:

1 Cup Banana (Chopped)

1 Cup Apple (Chopped)

1 Cup Frozen Mango (Chopped)

1 Tbsp. Turmeric Powder

1/4 Ginger Powder

200ml Coconut Milk

1-Cup Ice Cubes

Directions:

Blend everything and serve.

Nutrition:

Calories: 280 kcal,

Carbs: 34 g,

Fat: 8g,

Protein: 2 g.

Turmeric Almond Smoothie

Preparation Time: 5 minutes

Cooking Time: 0 minute

Servings: 2

Ingredients:

250ml Golden Milk

200ml Almond Milk

1/4 tbsp. Turmeric Powder

1/4 tbsp. Cinnamon Powder

1/2 tbsp. Vanilla Extract

2 Cups Chopped Banana

1 tbsp. Brown Sugar

1 Cup Ice Cubes

Directions:

Blend everything and serve.

Nutrition:

Calories:245 kcal,

Carbs: 43.6 g,

Fat: 7.1 g,

Protein: 5.5 g.

Green Smoothie

Preparation Time: 5 minutes

Cooking Time: 0 minute

Servings: 2

Ingredients:

250ml Almond Milk

100gm Frozen Spinach

1 Ripe Banana

1-Cup Ice Cube

1-Cup Chopped Frozen Green Apple

Directions:

Blend and serve with fruits.

Nutrition:

Calories:198 kcal

Carbs: 44 g

Fat: 1 g

Protein: 4 g

Choco Loco Tea Drink

Preparation Time: 10 minutes

Cooking Time: 0 minutes

Servings: 1

Ingredients:

1 1/2 cups boiling water

1 green tea bag

1 tbsp. cacao powder

1 tbsp. honey

¼ tsp cinnamon

½ cup almond milk

Directions:

In a large mug, add hot water and tea bag. Let it steep for 10 minutes.

Discard tea bag. Stir in honey, cinnamon and cacao powder. Mix well.

Stir in mint almond milk.

Serve and enjoy.

Nutrition:

Calories 152

Total Fat 2g

Saturated Fat 0g - Total Carbs 35g

Net Carbs 33g

Protein 2g - Sugar: 28g Fiber 2g Sodium 101mg

Potassium 189mg

Iced Matcha

Preparation Time: 10 minutes

Cooking Time: 0 minutes

Servings: 1

Ingredients:

½ cup hot water

1 teaspoon matcha tea powder

½ cup organic coconut milk (or whatever dairy/non-dairy drink you prefer)

1 teaspoon raw organic honey

Ice cubes

Directions:

In a large mug, add hot water and dissolve matcha powder. Mix well.

Mix in the rest of ingredients.

Serve and enjoy.

Nutrition:

Calories 298

Fat 29g

Carbs 13g

Protein 3g

Sugar: 10g

Fiber 3g

Sodium 21mg

Potassium 320mg

Turmeric-Spiced Coconut Milk Shake

Preparation Time: 10 minutes

Cooking Time: 0 minutes

Servings: 1

Ingredients:

½ tsp Turmeric Powder

¼ tsp ginger powder

¼ tsp cinnamon powder

2 tbsp. flaxseed, ground

1 cup water

1 cup coconut milk

Directions:

Add all ingredients in a blender.

Blend until smooth and creamy.

Serve and enjoy.

Nutrition:

Calories 266

Total Fat 17g

Carbs 19g

Protein 12g - Sugar: 13g

Fiber 6g

Sodium 116mg Potassium 526mg

Pomegranate-Avocado Smoothie

Preparation Time: 10 minutes

Cooking Time: 0 minutes

Servings: 1

Ingredients:

½ cup spinach

½ cup ice

½ tsp vanilla extract

½ tbsp. honey

½ cup Pomegranate Juice

¼ cup Greek Yogurt

½ Avocado, peeled

Directions:

Add all ingredients in a blender.

Blend until smooth and creamy.

Serve and enjoy.

Nutrition:

Calories 295

 Total Fat 15g

Carbs 36g

Protein 7g

Sugar: 27g - Fiber 7g

Sodium 46mg

Potassium 906mg

Oats, Flaxseeds and Banana Smoothie

Preparation Time: 10 minutes

Cooking Time: 0 minutes

Servings: 1

Ingredients:

½ cup of ice

1 tsp honey

2 tsp flaxseeds

¼ cup 100% whole grain rolled oats

1/2 cup Greek Yogurt, plain

½ cup almond milk

½ banana, peeled

¼ cup kale, shredded and stems discarded

Directions:

Add all ingredients in a blender.

Blend until smooth and creamy.

Serve and enjoy.

Nutrition:

Calories 305

Total Fat 10g

Total Carbs 54g Protein 11g

Sugar: 30g Fiber 8g Sodium 147mg

Potassium 703mg

Berry Red Smoothie

Preparation Time: 10 minutes

Cooking Time: 0 minutes

Servings: 1

Ingredients:

2 tbsp. cocoa powder

2 dried and pitted dates, sliced

1 cup almond milk

1 frozen banana

4 medium hulled strawberries

¾ cup raw red beets

Directions:

Add all ingredients in a blender.

Blend until smooth and creamy.

Serve and enjoy.

Nutrition:

Calories 377

Total Fat 10g

Carbs 69

Protein 13g

Sugar: 45g

Fiber 11g

Sodium 188mg

Potassium 1514mg

Pineapple Banana-Oat Smoothie

Preparation Time: 10 minutes

Cooking Time: 0 minutes

Servings: 1

Ingredients:

5-6 ice cubes

¼ tsp coconut extract

½ cup diced pineapple, fresh frozen

½ banana, frozen

1 container of 5.3oz nonfat Greek yogurt

¼ cup quick-cooking oats

1 cup almond milk

Directions:

In a microwave-safe cup, microwave on high for 2.5 minutes the 1 cup almond milk and ¼ cup oats.

Once oats are cooked, add 2 ice cubes to cool it down quick and mix.

Then pour the rest of the ingredients in a blender and puree until mixture is smooth and creamy along with the slightly cold cooked oats.

Nutrition:

Calories 255

Total Fat 4g

Saturated Fat 2g

Total Carbs 45g - Net Carbs 41g

Protein 14g

Sugar: 29g

Fiber 4g - Sodium 123mg - Potassium 751mg

Pineapple-Lettuce Smoothie

Preparation Time: 10 minutes

Cooking Time: 0 minutes

Servings: 2

Ingredients:

¼ tsp ground cinnamon

3 dates

1 banana, peeled and frozen

2 ½ cups fresh orange juice

2 ½ cups pineapple juice

½ apple

¼ cup red leaf lettuce

½ cup Romaine lettuce

Directions:

Add all ingredients in a blender.

Blend until smooth and creamy.

Serve and enjoy.

Nutrition:

Calories 352

Total Fat 1.2g

Carbs 88g

Protein 4.5g

Sugar: 65g

Fiber 7g Sodium 7mg Potassium 1206mg

Spiced Carrot Smoothie

Preparation Time: 10 minutes

Cooking Time: 0 minutes

Servings: 1

Ingredients:

1 cup spinach, optional

½ tsp ground cinnamon

½ tsp vanilla extract

1 banana, frozen

1 cup carrot, peeled and halved

1 cup almond milk

3 tbsp. raisins

Directions:

Add all ingredients in a blender.

Blend until smooth and creamy.

Serve and enjoy.

Nutrition:

Calories 274

Total Fat 3g

Carbs 53g

Protein 11g

Sugar: 34g

Fiber 8g

Sodium 209mg

Potassium 1329mg

Mango, Cucumber and Spinach Smoothie

Preparation Time: 10 minutes

Cooking Time: 0 minutes

Servings: 1

Ingredients:

1 cup water

1 cup orange juice, fresh

3 cups baby spinach

1 cup frozen mango, cubed and deseeded

2 apples, cored and chopped roughly

1 cucumber, ends removed and chopped roughly

Directions:

Add all ingredients in a blender.

Blend until smooth and creamy.

Serve and enjoy.

Nutrition:

Calories 455

Total Fat 2g

Carbs 111g

Protein 8g

Sugar: 84g

Fiber 15g

Sodium 90mg

Potassium 1885mg

Grape-Avocado Smoothie

Preparation Time: 10 minutes

Cooking Time: 0 minutes

Servings: 1

Ingredients:

1 tbsp. lime juice, fresh

2 tbsp. avocado

6oz Greek yogurt, plain

15 pcs red or green grapes

1 pear, peeled, cored and chopped

2 cups packed spinach leaves

Directions:

Add all ingredients in a blender.

Blend until smooth and creamy.

Serve and enjoy.

Nutrition:

Calories 243Total Fat 3g

Carbs 37g

Protein 20g

Sugar: 26g

Fiber 7g Sodium 111mg Potassium 949mg

Spiced Pumpkin Smoothie

Preparation Time: 10 minutes

Cooking Time: 0 minutes

Servings: 1

Ingredients:

Ice, optional

Pinch of nutmeg

½ tsp ginger

1 tsp cinnamon

1 small frozen banana

½ cup pureed pumpkin

1 tbsp. chia seeds

¼ cup rolled oats

1 cup almond milk

Directions:

Overnight or for an hour, soak chia seeds and oats in almond milk. This will give your smoothie a finer consistency.

Then, place all the ingredients in your food processor and blend ingredients until you get a smooth consistency.

Nutrition:

Calories 348

Total Fat 11g Carbs 61g Protein 15g

Sugar: 28g Fiber 9g Sodium 109mg

Potassium 1238mg

Almond and Pear Smoothie

Preparation Time: 10 minutes

Cooking Time: 0 minutes

Servings: 1

Ingredients:

2-3 dates, optional

¼ tsp ground cinnamon

1 tbsp. unsalted almond butter

½ cup almond milk

½ pear, deseeded

1 banana, frozen

Directions:

Add all ingredients in a blender.

Blend until smooth and creamy.

Serve and enjoy.

Nutrition:

Calories 341

Total Fat 11g

Saturated Fat 0.8g

Total Carbs 62g

Net Carbs 53g

Protein 6g

Sugar: 41g Fiber 9g

Sodium 88mg Potassium 826mg

Berry Nutty Smoothie

Preparation Time: 10 minutes

Cooking Time: 0 minutes

Servings: 1

Ingredients:

1 cup frozen mix berries

½ cup almond milk

¼ cup raw cashews

¼ cup quick-cooking oats

1 cup packed Romaine lettuce

¼ cup packed Swiss chard, packed, chopped and stems discarded

Ice cubes or cold water - optional

Directions:

Add all ingredients in a blender.

Blend until smooth and creamy.

Serve and enjoy.

Nutrition:

Calories 269

Total Fat 10g

Carbs 43g

Protein 6g

Sugar: 25g

Fiber 7g

Sodium 114mg Potassium 459mg

Mango Juice

Preparation Time: 10 minutes

Cooking Time: 0 minute

Servings: 4

Ingredients:

1 cups of cubed ripe mango

2 cup of orange juice

1 cup of water

½ inch of ginger

5 mint leaves

Directions:

Add all the ingredients to a blender and blend until smooth.

Serve immediately. Can be served with ice.

Nutrition:

Calcium: 14mg

Dietary Fiber: 1.1g

Protein: 1.3g

Potassium: 334mg

Sodium: 4mg

Sugar 16g

Carbs 19.5g

Fats: 0.1g

Calories: 83

Cucumber Celery Juice

Preparation Time: 5 minutes

Cooking Time: 0 minute

Servings: 2

Ingredients:

2 cups of cubed cucumber

2 cups of sliced celery sticks

1 cup of ice cubes

1 cup of water

½ inch of ginger

Salt and black pepper to taste

Directions:

Add all the ingredients to a blender and blend until smooth.

Serve immediately.

Nutrition:

Fiber: 1.3g

Protein: 0.4g

Potassium: 85mg

Sodium: 60mg

Sugar: .9g

Carbs: 4.2g

Fat: 0.1g

Calories: 19

CHAPTER 12: SAUCES, CONDIMENTS AND DRESSING

Tofu-Basil Sauce

Preparation Time: 10 minutes

Cooking Time: 0 minutes

Servings: 2 cups

Ingredients:

1 (12-ounce) package silken tofu

½ cup chopped fresh basil

2 garlic cloves, lightly crushed

½ cup almond butter

1 tablespoon fresh lemon juice

1 teaspoon salt

¼ teaspoon freshly ground black pepper

Directions:

In a blender or food processor, combine the tofu, basil, garlic, almond butter, lemon juice, salt, and pepper.

Process until smooth. If too thick, thin with a bit of water.

Refrigerate in an airtight container for up to 5 days.

Nutrition:

Calories: 120

Total fat: 10g

Total Carbohydrates: 5g

Sugar: 1g

Fiber: 2g

Protein: 6g

Sodium: 290mg

Apple Chutney

Preparation Time: 10 minutes

Cooking Time: 10 minutes

Servings: 2 cups

Ingredients:

1 tablespoon almond oil

4 apples, peeled, cored, and diced

1 small onion, diced

½ cup white raisins (optional)

1 tablespoon apple cider vinegar

1 tablespoon honey

1 teaspoon ground cinnamon

½ teaspoon ground cardamom

½ teaspoon ground ginger

½ teaspoon salt

Directions:

In a medium saucepan, heat the oil over low heat.

Add the apples, onion, raisins (if using), vinegar, honey, cinnamon, cardamom, ginger, and salt.

Cook briefly, just until the apples begin to release their juices.

Bring to a simmer, cover, and cook until the apples are tender 5 to 10 minutes.

Allow to cool completely before serving.

Nutrition:

Calories: 120

Total fat: 2g

Total carbohydrates: 24g

Sugar: 18

Fiber: 3g

Protein: 1g

Sodium: 150mg

Zesty Spice Rub

Preparation Time: 10 minutes

Cooking Time: 0 minutes

Servings: ½ cup

Ingredients:

1 tablespoon ground turmeric

1 tablespoon ground ginger

1 tablespoon ground fennel seed

1 tablespoon coconut sugar (optional)

2 teaspoons salt

2 teaspoons onion powder

1 teaspoon garlic powder

1 teaspoon paprika

½ teaspoon freshly ground black pepper

Directions:

Combine all the ingredients in a small bowl and mix well.

Store in an airtight container for up to 12 months.

Nutrition:

Calories: 20

Total carbohydrates: 5g

Fiber: 2g

Protein: 1g

Sodium: 1,160mg

Ginger-Turmeric Dressing

Preparation Time: 10 minutes

Cooking Time: 0 minutes

Servings: 1 ½ cups

Ingredients:

1 cup extra-virgin olive oil

¼ cup apple cider vinegar

½ teaspoon dijon mustard

1 garlic clove, sliced

½ teaspoon minced fresh ginger root

1 teaspoon salt

½ teaspoon ground turmeric

¼ teaspoon ground coriander

¼ teaspoon freshly ground black pepper

Directions:

In a blender or food processor, combine all the ingredients and process until smooth. Refrigerate in an airtight container for up to a week.

Nutrition:

Calories: 160

Total fat: 18g

Sodium: 200mg

Lemony Mustard Dressing

Preparation Time: 10 minutes

Cooking Time: 0 minutes

Servings: 1 ½ cups

Ingredients:

1 cup extra-virgin olive oil

¼ cup fresh lemon juice

1 tablespoon honey

1 teaspoon dijon mustard

1 shallot, sliced

1 teaspoon grated lemon zest

1 teaspoon salt

¼ teaspoon pepper

Directions:

In a blender or food processor, combine the olive oil, lemon juice, honey, dijon, shallot, lemon zest, salt, and pepper.

Process until smooth.

Refrigerate in an airtight container for up to 5 days.

Nutrition:

Calories: 180

Total fat: 20g

Total carbohydrates: 2g

Sugar: 2g

Sodium: 220mg

Lemon-Ginger Honey

Preparation Time: 10 minutes

Cooking Time: 0 minute

Servings: 1 cup

Ingredients:

1 cup water

¼ cup fresh lemon juice

2 tablespoons honey

2 teaspoons grated fresh ginger root

Directions:

Combine all the ingredients in an airtight jar and shake until the honey is dissolved.

Refrigerate for 24 hours before using so the ginger can permeate the mixture.

Store in the refrigerator up to a week.

Nutrition:

Calories: 20

Total carbohydrates: 5g

Sugar: 4g

Walnut Pesto

Preparation Time: 10 minutes

Cooking Time: 0 minute

Servings: 8

Ingredients:

½ Cup walnuts

¼ cup extra-virgin olive oil

4 garlic cloves, minced

1 cup baby spinach

¼ cup basil leaves

½ teaspoon sea salt

Directions:

In a blender or food processor, combine the walnuts, olive oil, garlic, spinach, basil, and salt.

Pulse for 15 to 20 (1-second) bursts, or until everything is finely chopped.

Nutrition:

Calories: 106

Total Fat: 11g

Total Carbs: 1g

Sugar: 1g

Fiber: 1g

Protein: 2g

Sodium: 120mg

Spinach Presto

Preparation Time: 10 minutes

Cooking Time: 0 minute

Servings: 4

Ingredients:

1 cup fresh baby spinach

½ cup fresh basil leaves

¼ cup pine nuts

¼ cup extra-virgin olive oil

4 garlic cloves, minced

2 ounces parmesan cheese, grated

½ teaspoon sea salt

Directions:

In a blender or food processor, combine the spinach, basil, pine nuts, olive oil, garlic, parmesan cheese, and salt.

Pulse for 15 to 20 (1-second) bursts, or until everything is finely chopped.

Keep refrigerated in a tightly sealed container for 5 days.

Mayonnaise

Preparation Time: 10 minutes

Cooking Time: 0 minute

Servings: 1 cup

Ingredients:

1 egg yolk

1 tablespoon apple cider vinegar

½ teaspoon Dijon mustard

Pinch sea salt

¾ cup extra-virgin olive oil

Directions:

In a blender or food processor, combine the egg yolk, cider vinegar, mustard, and salt. Turn on the blender or food processor and while it's running, remove the top spout. Carefully, working one drip at a time to start, drip in the olive oil.

After about 15 drops, continue to run the processor and add the oil in a thin stream until emulsified.

You may adjust the amount of oil to adjust the thickness. The more oil you add, the thicker the mayonnaise will be.

Keep this refrigerated for up to 4 days in a tightly sealed container.

Nutrition:

Calories: 169

Total Fat: 20g

Total Carbs: <1g

Sugar: 0g Fiber: 0g Protein: <1g

Sodium: 36mg

Stir-Fry Sauce

Preparation Time: 5 minutes

Cooking Time: 0 minute

Servings: 4

Ingredients:

¼ Cup low-sodium soy sauce

3 garlic cloves, minced

Juice of 2 limes

1 tablespoon grated fresh ginger

1 tablespoon arrowroot powder

Directions:

In a small bowl, whisk together the soy sauce, garlic, lime juice, ginger, and arrowroot powder.

Nutrition:

Calories: 24

Total Carbs: 4g

Sugar: 2g

Protein: 1g

Sodium: 887mg

Ginger-Teriyaki Sauce

Preparation Time: 5 minutes

Cooking Time: 0 minute

Ingredients:

¼ Cup low-sodium soy sauce

¼ cup pineapple juice

2 tablespoons packed brown sugar

1 tablespoon grated fresh ginger

1 tablespoon arrowroot powder or cornstarch

1 teaspoon garlic powder

Directions:

In a small bowl, whisk the soy sauce, pineapple juice, brown sugar, ginger, arrowroot powder, and garlic powder.

Keep refrigerated in a tightly sealed container for up to 5 days.

Nutrition:

Calories: 41

Total Carbs: 10g

Sugar: 7g

Protein: 1g

Sodium: 882mg

Garlic Aioli

Preparation Time: 5 minutes

Cooking Time: 0 minute

Servings: 4

Ingredients:

½ Cup anti-inflammatory mayonnaise (here)

3 garlic cloves, finely minced

Directions:

In a small bowl, whisk the mayonnaise and garlic to combine.

Keep refrigerated in a tightly sealed container for up to 4 days.

Nutrition:

Calories: 169

Total Fat: 20g

Total Carbs: <1g

Sugar: 0g

Fiber: 0g

Protein: <1g

Sodium: 36mg

Raspberry Vinaigrette

Preparation Time: 5 minutes

Cooking Time: 0 minutes

Servings: 8

Ingredients:

¾ Cup extra-virgin olive oil

¼ cup apple cider vinegar

¼ cup fresh raspberries, crushed with the back of a spoon

3 garlic cloves, finely minced

½ teaspoon sea salt

⅛ teaspoon freshly ground black pepper

Directions:

In a small bowl, whisk the olive oil, cider vinegar, raspberries, garlic, salt, and pepper

Keep refrigerated in a tightly sealed container for up to 5 days.

Nutrition:

Calories: 167

Total Fat: 19g

Total Carbs: <1g

Sugar: 0g

Fiber: 0g

Protein: <1g

Sodium: 118mg

Lemon-Ginger Vinaigrette

Preparation Time: 5 minutes

Cooking Time: 0 minute

Servings: 8

Ingredients:

¾ Cup extra-virgin olive oil

¼ cup freshly squeezed lemon juice

1 tablespoon grated fresh ginger

1 garlic clove, minced

½ teaspoon sea salt

⅛ Teaspoon freshly ground black pepper

Directions:

In a small bowl, whisk the olive oil, lemon juice, ginger, garlic, salt, and pepper

Keep refrigerated in a tightly sealed container for up to 5 days.

Nutrition:

Calories: 167

Total Fat: 19g

Total Carbs: <1g

Sugar: 0g

Fiber: 0g

Protein: <1g

Sodium: 118mg

Peanut Sauce

Preparation Time: 5 minutes

Cooking Time: 0 minute

Servings: 8

Ingredients:

1 cup lite coconut milk

¼ cup creamy peanut butter

¼ cup freshly squeezed lime juice

3 garlic cloves, minced

2 tablespoons low-sodium soy sauce, or gluten-free soy sauce, or tamari

1 tablespoon grated fresh ginger

Directions:

In a blender or food processor, process the coconut milk, peanut butter, lime juice, garlic, soy sauce, and ginger until smooth.

Keep refrigerated in a tightly sealed container for up to 5 days.

Nutrition:

Calories: 143

Total Fat: 11g

Total Carbs: 8g

Sugar: 2g

Fiber: 1g

Protein: 6g

Sodium: 533mg

Garlic Ranch Dressing

Preparation Time: 5 minutes

Cooking Time: 0 minute

Servings: 8

Ingredients:

1 cup nonfat plain greek yogurt

1 garlic clove, minced

2 tablespoons chopped, fresh chives

¼ cup chopped, fresh dill

Zest of 1 lemon

½ teaspoon sea salt

⅛ teaspoon freshly cracked black pepper

Directions:

In a small bowl, whisk together the yogurt, garlic, chives, dill, lemon zest, salt, and pepper.

Keep refrigerated in a tightly sealed container for up to 5 days.

Nutrition:

Calories: 17

Total Fat: 0g;

Total Carbs: 3g

Sugar: 2g

Fiber: 0g

Protein: 2g Sodium: 140mg

Easy Garlicky Cherry Tomato Sauce

Preparation Time: 5 Minutes

Cooking Time: 25 Minutes

Servings: 4

Ingredients:

¼ cup extra virgin olive oil

¼ thinly sliced garlic cloves

2 pounds organic cherry tomatoes

½ teaspoon dried oregano

1 teaspoon coconut sugar

¼ cup chopped fresh basil 1 teaspoon salt

Directions:

Heat oil in a large saucepan over medium heat.

Sauté the garlic for a minute until fragrant.

Add in the cherry tomatoes and season with salt, oregano, coconut sugar, and fresh basil.

Allow to simmer for 25 minutes until the tomatoes are soft and become a thick sauce.

Place in containers and store in the fridge until ready to use.

Nutrition:

Calories: 198 Cal

Fat: 6 g

Carbs: 37 g Protein: 3 g

Fiber: 5 g

Avocado Cilantro Detox Dressing

Preparation Time: 5 Minutes

Cooking Time: 0 minute

Servings: 3

Ingredients:

5 tablespoons lemon juice, freshly squeezed

1 clove of garlic, chopped

1 avocado, pitted and flesh scooped out

1 bunch cilantro, chopped

¼ teaspoon salt

¼ cup water

Directions:

Place all ingredients in a food processor and pulse until well combined.

Pulse until creamy.

Place in a lidded container and store in the fridge until ready to use.

Use on salads and sandwiches.

Nutrition:

Calories 114 Cal

Fat: 10 g

Carbs: 8 g

Protein: 2 g

Fiber: 5 g

Golden Turmeric Sauce

Preparation Time: 10 Minutes

Cooking Time: 15 Minutes

Servings: 4

Ingredients:

2 tablespoons coconut oil

2-inch piece ginger, peeled and minced

2 cloves of garlic, minced

2 cups white sweet potato, cubed

2 tablespoons turmeric powder

½ teaspoon ginger powder

¼ teaspoon cinnamon powder

2 cups coconut milk 1 onion, chopped

Juice from 1 lemon, freshly squeezed

1 cup water 1 ½ teaspoon salt

Directions:

Heat oil in a saucepan over medium flame.

Sauté the onion, ginger, and garlic until fragrant.

Add in the sweet potatoes, turmeric powder, ginger powder, and cinnamon powder.

Pour in water and season with salt. Bring to a boil for 10 minutes.

Once the potatoes are soft, place in a blender pulse until smooth.

Return the mixture into the saucepan.

Turn on the stove. Add in the coconut milk and lemon juice.

Allow to simmer for 5 minutes.

Store in lidded containers and put inside the fridge until ready to use.

Nutrition:

Calories: 172

Fat: 11g

Carbs: 15g

Protein: 5g

Fiber: 3g

Creamy Turmeric Dressing

Preparation Time: 5 Minutes

Cooking Time: 0 minute

Servings: 6

Ingredients:

½ cup tahini

½ cup olive oil

2 tablespoons lemon juice

2 teaspoons honey

Salt to taste

A dash of black pepper

Directions:

Mix all ingredients in a bowl until the mixture becomes creamy and smooth.

Store in lidded containers.

Put in the fridge until ready to use.

Nutrition:

Calories 286

Fat 29g

Carbs 7g

Protein 4g

Fiber: 2 g

CHAPTER 13: WEEKLY MEAL PLAN

13.1 First Week

Days	Breakfast	Lunch	Dinner	Snack
	Turmeric Oven Scrambled Eggs	Green Soup	Tasty Turkey Baked Balls	Chickpeas and Pepper Hummus
	Breakfast Oatmeal	Buckwheat Noodle Soup	Sprouts & Slices In Wheat Wrap	Lemony Chickpeas Dip
	Blueberry Smoothie	Zoodles	Feta-Filled & Tomato-Topped Turkey Burger Bites	Chili Nuts
	Breakfast Porridge	Chickpea Curry	Simply Sautéed Chinese Chicken	Protein Bars
	Quinoa And Asparagus Mushroom Frittata	Ratatouille	Zesty Zucchini & Chicken In Classic Santa Fe Stir-Fry	Red Pepper Muffins
	Cherry Spinach Smoothie	Herbed Baked Salmon	Crispy Cheese-Crusted Fish Fillet	Nuts And Seeds Mix
	Tropical Carrot Ginger And Turmeric Smoothie	Carrot Soup	Ambrosial Avocado & Salmon Salad In Lemon-Dressed Layers	Tortilla Chips

13.2 Second Week

Days	Breakfast	Lunch	Dinner	Snack
	Golden Milk Chia Pudding	Lentil Soup	Sautéed Shrimp Jambalaya Jumble	Kale Chips
	No-Bake Turmeric Protein Donuts	Miso Broiled Salmon	Baked Buffalo Cauliflower Chunks	Potato Chips
	Choco-Nana Pancakes	Broccoli Cauliflower Salad	Cool Garbanzo and Spinach Beans	Peach Dip
	Sweet Potato	Spinach Salad	Lemony Garlic	Cereal

	Cranberry Breakfast Bars	With Beans	Shrimp	Mix
	Savory Breakfast Pancakes	Goat Cheese & Bell Pepper Salad	Coconut and Hazelnut Chilled Glass	Eggplant, Olives And Basil Salad
	Scrambled Eggs With Smoked Salmon	Green Soup	Coriander Greens With Zucchini Sauté	Fresh Tomato, Onion and Jalapeno Pepper Salsa
	Raspberry Grapefruit Smoothie	Buckwheat Noodle Soup	Walnuts and Asparagus Delight	Fresh Veggie Bars

13.3 Third Week

Days	Breakfast	Lunch	Dinner	Snack
	Breakfast Burgers With Avocado Buns	Zoodles	Tasty Turkey Baked Balls	Green Beans And Avocado With Chopped Cilantro
	Buckwheat And Chia Seed Porridge	Chickpea Curry	Sprouts & Slices In Wheat Wrap	Parsnip Fries
	Turmeric Oven Scrambled Eggs	Ratatouille	Feta-Filled & Tomato-Topped Turkey Burger Bites	Spinach Chips
	Breakfast Oatmeal	Herbed Baked Salmon	Simply Sautéed Chinese Chicken	Fruit Salsa
	Blueberry Smoothie	Carrot Soup	Zesty Zucchini & Chicken In Classic Santa Fe Stir-Fry	Cauliflower Hummus
	Breakfast Porridge	Lentil Soup	Crispy Cheese-Crusted Fish Fillet	Chickpeas and

				Pepper Hummus
	Quinoa And Asparagus Mushroom Frittata	Miso Broiled Salmon	Ambrosial Avocado & Salmon Salad In Lemon-Dressed Layers	Lemony Chickpeas Dip

13.4 Fourth Week

Days	Breakfast	Lunch	Dinner	Snack
	Cherry Spinach Smoothie	Broccoli Cauliflower Salad	Sautéed Shrimp Jambalaya Jumble	Chili Nuts
	Tropical Carrot Ginger And Turmeric Smoothie	Spinach Salad With Beans	Baked Buffalo Cauliflower Chunks	Protein Bars
	Golden Milk Chia Pudding	Goat Cheese & Bell Pepper Salad	Cool Garbanzo and Spinach Beans	Red Pepper Muffins
	No-Bake Turmeric Protein Donuts	Green Soup	Lemony Garlic Shrimp	Nuts And Seeds Mix
	Choco-Nana Pancakes	Buckwheat Noodle Soup	Coconut and Hazelnut Chilled Glass	Tortilla Chips
	Sweet Potato Cranberry Breakfast Bars	Zoodles	Coriander Greens With Zucchini Sauté	Kale Chips
	Savory Breakfast Pancakes	Chickpea Curry	Walnuts and Asparagus Delight	Potato Chips

CHAPTER 14: VITAMINS

Taking anti-inflammatory vitamins can reduce swelling, pains, and redness. When you have an accident or get a cold, the natural reaction of our bodies is to inflame the injured area to address off any threats around the body defense mechanism. The usual response can heal diseases, infections, and injuries. Without inflammation, soreness is experienced in the affected area.

14.1 How to Reduce Inflammation using Vitamins

Taking vitamin, supplements, or medications is the best method to relieve inflammation, although it all begins from your diet. Adding anti-inflammatory foods in your daily diet is the foundation of preventing inflammation. These include; leafy green vegetables, fruits which might be high in antioxidants, healthy fats, fish, and nuts. Try to avoid unhealthy food and refined sugars; they worsen inflammation. Surprisingly, drinking your coffee may prevent inflammation. Coffee contains polyphenols and other anti-inflammatory compounds. It is also an incredible acidic drink. However, if you add milk and sugar, the coffee can trigger inflammation.

If you suffer from digestive issues, gastritis or ulcers, it's advisable to avoid inflammation. Try to incorporate gentle exercise and yoga alongside your diet plan to keep it away. In one study, the participants performed a three-month yoga retreat and their inflammation levels got tested. After the period, they noted a massive decrease in their inflammatory markers and the metabolic risk factors. When you calm the body and your brain, it reduces chronic inflammation. Lastly, including supplements and vitamins in your diet reduces inflammation. Remember, before the doctor prescribes any medication, it's essential to inform them that you are taking anti-inflammation and vitamins.

14.2 The Anti-inflammatory Vitamins

When you have a scratched knee, swelling around the cut area is a healthy thing, which signifies that the body's defense mechanism is battling germs from the tissue. Also, developing a swollen ankle once you sprain proofs healing. However, if you cannot see or feel the condition, it can prolong and trigger diabetes, cancer, heart diseases, and other autoimmune, including psoriasis and arthritis rheumatoid. There are different vitamins with the anti-inflammatory potential. Vitamin intake can be measured accurately and controlled. Eating food rich in vitamins is an added advantage. However, if you are overweight, this proper diet will help you to drop some weight-reducing chances of inflammation. Remember, taking a hefty dose of the particular vitamin may be risky; that's why you should seek the doctor's advice before thinking about nutritional vitamins. Researchers have identified vitamins that contain anti-inflammatory compounds. They could be administered in supplement form, or natural (from the food you consume.)

Here is a list of the vitamins that have anti-inflammatory properties and foods which are abundant options for these vitamins:

Vitamin A

Vitamin A is vital for maintaining the body's functioning and regulating defense mechanisms. Its deficiency is common, and it increases the risks of acquiring infections for both males and females. It's also an anti-inflammatory agent that reduces inflammatory conditions, including acne vulgaris and precancerous. Study shows that vitamin A can prevent the defense mechanism from reacting, causing inflammation. It exists in two forms; Beta-carotene and vitamin A.

Beta-carotene is a pro-vitamin that converts vitamin A in the body, an antioxidant protecting the body against poisons. Both types help in reducing inflammation. The foods containing vitamin A are varieties of leafy vegetables, including kales, spinach, collard greens, and carrots.

Vitamin B

Low amounts of vitamin B can result in chronic inflammation in our systems. However, do not over-consume the vitamin because new studies have shown a link between chronic inflammation with vitamins found in foods like legumes, vegetables, and liver. A study signifies that vitamin B6 causes high chronic inflammation in your blood. However, swelling after an accident is a symbol of a temporary inflammation that indicates that the immune system is actively preventing the problem. Chronic inflammation is a hazard to health factors resulting in a stroke, diabetes type 2 symptoms, and heart diseases. A high C-reactive-protein results in low vitamin B6 that causes inflammation and autoimmune diseases such as rheumatism. Foods that contain plenty of vitamin B include; poultry, liver, dark leafy greens, black-eyed peas, tuna, bell peppers, asparagus, mushroom, and kale. An Italian study also shows that when small doses of folic acid supplements are taken persistently, they can reduce the condition.

Vitamin C

Inflammation is a silent killer and prolonged chronic inflammation causes degenerative diseases like heart diseases, diabetes, and obesity. There is a link between age-related blindness in adults 50 plus and chronic inflammation. High levels of vitamin C in our systems will massively lower inflammation. Consuming fruits can reduce its danger by 25 percent. Vitamin C maintains healthy and functioning defense mechanisms. Also, it eliminates free-radicals that cause inflammation. Vitamin C is just like B since it lowers the C-reactive proteins. Although vitamin supplements are vital in inflammation, it's good to get them from your diet plan.

Vitamin D

A high percentage of people have vitamin D deficiency. A direct link exists between various inflammation diseases and a lower vitamin D. Furthermore, research shows that better vitamin D levels can reduce inflammation. There are molecular reasons behind vitamin D's abilities to fight inflammation. People with lower amounts of vitamin D can benefit from vitamin supplements. Sun is a natural source of vitamin D, although it can be inadequate, especially to people who do not access plenty of it. We can find Vitamin K2 in organ meats, milk, fish, and yolks. However, if you feel like your levels of the vitamin have dropped, you can contact your doctor.

Vitamin E

It's an antioxidant that reduces and prevents inflammation. It can be naturally from nuts (such as sunflower and almonds) and vegetables and fruit full of vitamin E (like avocado and spinach.)Vitamin E is an essential vitamin required for the proper functioning of several body parts. The vitamin can also prevent heart diseases, inflammation, improve eye health, boost immune function, and lowering the potential risks of cancer. However, its benefit varies, and the supplement may not suit everyone.

Vitamin K

Vitamin K enhances blood clotting, bone health, and slows up the inflammatory markers. Although the vitamin is crucial to our bones, several people do not get it from their diets. Men are advised to take 120 mg daily and females about 90 mg. However, the daily intake for infants and children is lower than that of adults. It exists as Vitamin K2 and K1. Vitamin K2 could be found in liver, eggs, and chicken, while vitamin K1 can be obtained from leafy vegetables like kales, cabbages, and spinach.

CHAPTER 15: INTERMITTENT FASTING

15.1 Combination of Intermittent Fasting and Anti-Inflammatory Diet

When it comes to maximizing the effects of the anti-inflammatory diet, one step that many people find effective is to combine it with the habit of intermittent fasting to supercharge the effectiveness of both. This is due to the fact that intermittent fasting naturally serves to stabilize both glucose and blood sugar levels while naturally decreasing inflammation at the same time. If you do decide to go down this route, however, it is important that you give your body plenty of time to transition to the anti-inflammatory diet first, especially if you formerly consumed large amounts of processed foods. After about a month of following the anti-inflammatory diet, you should be ready to add in intermittent fasting as well.

15.2 Intermittent Fasting Benefits

Building muscle and losing weight are only two of the many benefits that fasting intermittently can lead to. It can also help you to find extra time in a busy schedule as you will find you suddenly don't have to worry about finding time for breakfast every single day. What's more, you will be surprised how much extra money not having to worry about breakfast actually saves you in the long run, even when you factor in the extra amount you are eating for the remaining meals as well. While giving up on breakfast might sound difficult, once new habits begin to form, it will seem like the most natural thing in the world.

Aside from the ancillary benefits, intermittent fasting will also literally help you live longer as being in a prolonged fasting state causes your body to divert extra energy to improving core biological functions as this state sends out emergency signals similar to those that are sent out when your body is starving. A fasting state is quite different from starving, however, and by simply skipping breakfast, you soon won't feel that much hungrier come lunchtime once your body has adapted.

Additional medical benefits include a decrease in the odds of contracting cardiovascular disease and cancer as well as a decreased risk of stroke. It is even known to lessen the aftereffects of chemotherapy. In fact, decreasing your daily calorie count by just 15 percent is known to improve your glucose tolerance and lowers blood pressure, improves oxidative resistance, kidney function, and reproductive effectiveness.

While the reasons behind these benefits aren't entirely clear, it is likely due in part to the fact that intermittent fasting is known to decrease stress while at the same time making your body more resistant to many of the common effects of stress. This is especially true when it comes to organ and digestive tract health. It also improves how your mitochondria work, which makes them utilize energy more efficiently and leave you open to less oxidation based damage.

Furthermore, traditional intermittent fasting, as well as to alternate-day fasting, are medically approved ways of minimizing the risk of developing type 2 diabetes in those who are already suffering from pre-diabetes.

Both of these types of fasting are known to help glucose levels return to normal in as little as 12 months. This benefit can be negated, of course, if the practitioners of intermittent fasting use the fact that they are fasting as an excuse to eat anything and everything during the periods they are not dieting strictly. This is folly, however, as the best way to see long term results is to not treat fasting as something special and to instead think of it as just another part of your daily routine.

While there is plenty of real health benefits listed above, what many people ultimately find that they enjoy about intermittent fasting the most is the fact that it is just so simple and easy to use. So easy to use, in fact, that studies show that even those who were otherwise considered extremely overweight and had trouble dieting routinely were able to stick with it for 3 months or more, much longer than they were with any other type of more restrictive diet by a power of three or more.

Even better, while on the intermittent diet, these individuals saw just as much average weight loss as anyone else. Perhaps, the best data of all is that a year after the study completed, those who had started with intermittent fasting had managed to lose the most weight overall.

15.3 Types of Intermittent Fasting

The 16/8 Method: With this method, you are required to fast for 14 to 16 hours each day, and then the remainder of the day, you are technically able to eat whatever you would like. With this eating window, you still have enough time to eat two or three meals without too many issues, so it is still easy to fit this eating schedule into your day without feeling restricted.

This is a really easy method to follow, especially if you pick the right hours to do your fasting. For example, simply stop eating supper at around 8 pm and do not have any late-night snacks. When you get up the next day, you will skip breakfast and start eating around 12 pm. This will put you into a 16-hour fast.

The biggest issue that comes with this option is that some people feel hungry when they wake up in the morning or they have breakfast as part of their morning routine. If you like to eat breakfast, just stop eating around 5 pm and have breakfast at 9 am. You must be careful not to take any late-night snacks while you are on this plan, but it is much easier compared to some of the other options you may choose.

The 5/2 Method: This is another popular method of intermittent fasting that involves regularly eating for five days during the week while limiting the intake of calories to around 500-600 during the remaining two days. During the two fasting days, the recommended calorie intake for men and women is 600 and 500 calories, respectively. For instance, you can eat regularly on other days, and limit your intake to two small meals amounting to 250 calories each during say Mondays and Thursdays. The two fasting days should be non-consecutive.

The 5:2 diet plan is pretty accommodating and flexible with limited restrictions. You can pick when you want to eat and when you would like to fast depending on a schedule. It is more flexible compared to other methods when it comes to altering fasting and eating times. Some people may enjoy the idea of limiting or controlling their diet only twice a week.

Here comes the big catch now, especially for those who have not fasted before. Going off food for an entire day can be challenging if you are just getting started with intermittent fasting. This is more challenging for people who are required to perform demanding tasks throughout the day or those with families to look after (preparing meals for children).

Another flip side is that you have to caution against the trap of overeating after fasting for a long duration. Feeling ravenous after fasting for 24 hours may make you overeat; this may not really support your weight loss goals.

Alternate day fasting: With this method, the faster does a partial fast every other day, eating a limited amount of food for one day and then a normal amount the next day, and so on.

Because there are seven days in the week and the diet follows a schedule by the weekday, the dieter uses three specific days of every week to do a partial fast. Dieters using this model commonly choose to diet on Mondays, Wednesdays, and Fridays.

On those days, the dieter consumes only one-fifth of the normal number of calories that he or she consumes on the other days. If you are a man, you likely take in about 2,500 calories per day. If you are a woman, you likely consume about 2,000 calories per day. Therefore, you would consume 500 or 400 calories on Mondays, Wednesdays, and Fridays, which can easily be done by drinking protein shakes.

Protein shakes are very filling and are also low in calories. High-protein foods and vegetables will also help you to fill up faster. The experts sometimes recommend protein shakes for just the first two weeks of the diet and real food from the third week onward as it is always preferable to anything processed, even if it is marketed as health food.

Working out is not advised on this program if you must work out while on this diet, do a lighter version of your regular workouts on the days that you eat normally.

This diet can effectively drop about 2.5 pounds of weight per week for dieters who cut their calorie intake between 20 and 35 percent, and this is done without the dieter feeling hungry or having to follow a difficult schedule. Additionally, dieting on alternate days never allows leptin levels to fall, which means that the body never stops losing the fat. The dieter must be careful not to binge eat on their off days. This is not a program aimed for beginners or those who only need a slight reduction in weight.

Fat Loss Forever: Fat Loss Forever is an intermittent fasting program that essentially takes the best of all worlds by incorporating ideas from different intermittent fasting programs.

Day 1: Cheat day. A cheat day is exactly what it sounds like. You can eat whatever you want! However, you need to keep what you eat within reason. Eating whatever you want doesn't necessarily mean that you should head straight for the pizza buffet and follow it up with a giant ice cream sundae. Try to keep what you eat within reason. Aim for a high protein intake with a lot of fruits and vegetables. Throw in some special things that you are craving just to make the plan a little bit more fun.

Day 2: Full fast day. Like a cheat day, a full fast day is exactly what it sounds like: you don't consume any calories. You must consume large quantities of water in order to stay hydrated.

Day 3: 16:8 fasting. This day follows a diet schedule that is very similar to lean gains in that you fast for 16 hours and eat for 8.

Day 4: Full fast day. Again, a full fast day is exactly what it sounds like. You won't eat anything.

Day 5: 16:8 fasting. Again, by the end of this day's 16-hour fast, you will have fasted for 36 hours.

Day 6: Warrior diet. On this day, you will follow the procedures that are associated with the warrior diet. You will start off the day with a piece of fruit and a no-carb, high-protein shake, and then fast until 9 pm. As in the warrior diet, you will consume all of the day's calories within a four-hour window. You may want to plan ahead so that this is on a day when you might plan to go out in the evenings. Having something to look forward to and being able to consume a large number of calories in a social setting will make this day's fast easier.

Day 7: Cheat day.

CHAPTER 16: HOW TO REDUCE INFLAMMATION IN YOUR BODY

16.1 What Causes Inflammation in the Body And How Do I Control It?

Inflammation in the body is really useful and is treated as a major aspect of the body's framework. It goes about as a layer between the external condition and the influenced territory; it also represses the disease to spread to other body parts. In the event that there is an occurrence of any damage or disease, we see redness and soreness around the influenced territory. This is on the grounds that; the WBCs (white platelets) are joined to the inward linings of veins around the influenced territory.

Then again, if due to any reason, if WBCs begin regarding solid cells as remote material, increasingly more of WBCs begin gathering at the internal linings, bringing about agony and overabundance of soreness. This outcomes in endless inflammation, which, if not controlled at before, stages can prompt difficult conditions like arthritis, psoriasis, etc.

In the wake of understanding what causes irritation, let us currently discover a successful method for controlling it.

The best and regular approach to have a tab on the body's irritation cycle is to accomplish elevated amounts of DHA omega-3 unsaturated fats. These are long-chain polyunsaturated fats, which are required by the body for its legitimate development and improvement. Studies have demonstrated that the body can change over DHA to a synthetic called resolvin D2 that has a property to respond with internal linings of veins to shape nitric oxide. This layer of nitric oxide hinders abundance of WBCs to join the internal linings of veins, and thus helps in diminishing inflammation.

In this manner, it is our enthusiasm to have high DHA levels. Be that as it may, since the body can't deliver DHA alone, we need to take express activities to incorporate high DHA sustenance sources in our everyday diet.

Cold-water fish like hoki, tuna, salmon, etc. Are the rich wellspring of DHA fats. In any case, in view of expanding water contamination, fish are additionally loaded with pollutions like mercury, lead and arsenic. Clearly, it's anything but a decent arrangement to lessen inflammation in the body at the expense of eating poisons.

This is the place fish oil enhancements come to help. They experience refining procedures to expel all the undesirable and destructive synthetic compounds from the oil and are consequently, useful for human utilization.

Since you realize what causes inflammation in the body and how you can control the equivalent, your subsequent stage ought to be investing some more energy in the web to discover a viable enhancement and begin taking it right away.

Perpetual Inflammation in the body is dangerous

You know when you have a sore throat and your lymph hubs are swollen? Your body has sent in the military of white platelets to wreck the encompassing tissue and improve. The issue comes when it doesn't quit obliterating the sound tissue and continues onward.

Specialists have connected inflammation in your body with illnesses of different types such as asthma, rheumatoid joint pain, coronary illness, considerably malignant growth and memory misfortune.

Studies demonstrate it is basic to your wellbeing and prosperity to control inflammation in the body.

You may consider inflammation in swollen joints from joint pain agony or the swelling encompassing a paper cut, however, inflammation can be inside where its not obvious.

Excited corridors cause plaque development and block up the entry, which adds to a heart assault. Moreover, inflammation in your cerebrum blocks up the neuron pathways, so the messages aren't clear or don't get sent–this can prompt Alzheimer's.

Inflammation begins as your body's barrier against damage or sickness. It's your body's method for mending you. However, when its work is done, the inflammation should stop. Chronic inflammation can cause long haul harm.

16.2 The Guide To Getting Rid Of Inflammation In Your Body

Many of us experience the ill effects of inflammation in our bodies and we should comprehend what inflammation truly is.

Inflammation is a procedure brought about by our bodies to shield us from unsafe diseases or infections. If you experience the ill effects of inflammation in your body, you will have encountered redness or torment. There are numerous reasons for inflammation. It can be intense or incessant, but whichever way, there are a few things that you can do to dispose of it. Along these lines, how about we begin examining how to lessen inflammation in the body.

Decreasing this issue in your body is certifiably, not a troublesome assignment. So as to do this, you should watch what you eat and practice normally. How about we talk about each in detail.

When attempting to stay away from inflammation in your body, you should diminish your admission of handled nourishment. All and any sort of handled nourishment will contain sustenance that builds the irritation level in your body. Additionally, attempting to maintain a strategic distance from sustenance that contains high measures of sugar can consequently anticipate the issue that you should eat vegetables and organic products.

Vegetables and natural products contain mitigating properties. These nourishments have demonstrated to diminish irritation in the whole body. It is proposed to expend the vegetables and natural products that are brilliant in shading.

Additionally, in your customary eating diet increment, the admission of omega-3 unsaturated fat. Omega-3 is generally found in various kinds of nuts and seeds. Accordingly, make sure to eat pecans or sesame seeds all the time. Research demonstrates that green tea and straightforward water can help keep this issue from happening. Green tea and water are referred to go about as cell reinforcements, and with normal use, they will limit the issue. Aside from watching what you eat, practicing has demonstrated to help in keeping this from occurring. With exercise, you will shed pounds, when you get in shape, the measure of weight on your joints will be less. The less weight on your joints will help forestall an inflammation issue. Nonetheless, you should guarantee that you normally practice for in any event for 40 minutes.

The earlier mentioned systems are best in assisting with inflammation in the body. In any case, you can take supplements that are wealthy in fish oil or nutrients. Alongside these enhancements, ordinary body back rubs have demonstrated to help in preventing this from occurring. These back rubs should be possible with oil or basic creams. You can keep warmed cushions on your body, which will absolutely help. Despite the fact that these methods work, they are not as compelling as the adjusting of the eating regimen and working out. In this way, when attempting to ensure the body, you ought to consistently select to control what you eat and practice normally. Keep in mind that regardless of what procedure you pick, you have to guarantee that you are steady with it. Inflammation is treatable just in the event that you are given.

16.3 How To Reduce Inflammation In The Body That Requires Your Attention?

You're savvy to think about how to decrease inflammation in the body. What's more, you're significantly more astute to proceed to do it. All things considered, inflammation is the number reason for death. Time magazine called it "the Silent Killer" and specialists concur. Constant inflammation is the hidden explanation behind all intents and purposes for each savage malady you can consider.

Alright, so you realize you have to do it. How?

The means are basic, however difficult. It will require some move in your reasoning. Some way of life changes. In any case, is it certifiably not a more drawn out, more beneficial life justified, despite all the trouble?

Basic to decreasing your inflammation is your eating routine and exercise. In case you're eating a lousy nourishment, a diet loaded up with refined flours and sugars, you're making inflammation in your body. At any rate, restorative research demonstrates that is what's valid for the vast majority.

The manifestations of inflammation, swelling, redness and throbbing can be occurring inside your body without you knowing it. They're a sign your invulnerable framework is lopsided.

Supplanting undesirable nourishments with a lot of foods grown from the ground and getting ordinary exercise will help diminish inflammation for some individuals.

And when you presume a nourishment hypersensitivity/affectability, you can remove the potential sustenance for three times a month and check whether that makes a difference. A few specialists prescribe the 'Base Diet' where you only eat fish, meat, vegetables and organic products for a month. The thought is you're not eating any cutting edge handled sustenance, including grains. For some, this might be your answer.

Conclusion

Congratulations on finishing this book! You have done your body a tremendous favor and are now well on your way to maintaining a healthy lifestyle!

After having read this book and worked through the four-week meal plan, you should now have a solid foundational understanding of what inflammation is, what kind of inflammation is desirable and what kind is not, the causes of the various types of inflammation and their respective symptoms, the various treatment options that are available for the different causes of inflammation, how the human body uses the foods in our diets, how those foods can either reduce or encourage inflammation, as well as how and why anti-inflammatory diets work.

While you should be feeling an improvement in your health over the past four weeks, it is important to your long-term success that you do not simply forget everything you have learned and revert back to your old habits. Remember that your genetic expression can change throughout your lifetime, which means that you can get better or worse depending on the chemical environment that you put your cells in. You are now on the path towards a healthy cellular environment and, therefore, the expression of your healthiest genes. If you continue to exercise the knowledge you have gained from this book and to keep a close eye on your diet, your health will steadily improve and may even lead to the resolution of some of your most concerning health issues.

Remember also that although your diet is perhaps the single most important controllable factor in determining the level of inflammation you experience—it is by no means the only factor.

Keep in mind that the human body needs about eight to nine hours of sleep per night so that it can rejuvenate itself for the following day. If you do not give your body the amount of sleep it requires each night, you are not only encouraging the inflammatory process, but you are also much more likely to make poor dietary choices, which, in turn, will also encourage the body's inflammatory process. This cycle will put your body in a constant state of damage control, which can ultimately result in chronic inflammation and all the health complications, which can result therefrom. For these same reasons, it is also important that you remember to relax by making a habit out of meditation or deep breathing exercises, as chronic stress can have similarly disastrous effects on your health and diet, as can the failure to get enough sleep.

Regular exercise is another important factor to keep in mind when trying to control your inflammation. Leading a life that is too sedentary will result in the deterioration and atrophy of your physical, mental, and emotional health. By getting in 20 minutes of physical activity each day, whether by taking a walk or going for a jog, your body will release chemicals that will improve your attitude, bring positive emotions, and strengthen the immune functions of your body. Your body will then be much better able to rid itself of environmental toxins, reduce the amount of inflammation it may be inclined to develop, and thereby encourage a generally healthy environment in which your best genes express themselves.

This book has shown you that when it comes to controlling inflammation, your diet is of the utmost importance and will, therefore, dramatically affect your health and lifestyle. The reverse is also true—your health and lifestyle will dramatically affect your diet. We can see, then, that when all is said and done, preventing or reducing chronic inflammation boils down to general lifestyle choices. Maintaining a healthy diet is the first step in making healthy lifestyle choices, and by working through this book, you have taken the first step towards maintaining that healthy diet. Keep up the good work, and constantly be on the lookout for ways to encourage your genes to respond positively to your environment—your body and mind will thank you for it!

I hope you have found this book useful, and I sincerely wish you success on the journey you have undertaken towards living a long, happy, and healthy life!

CPSIA information can be obtained
at www.ICGtesting.com
Printed in the USA
LVHW061552200621
690710LV00005B/255